THE JOHN HENRY HEALTH EQUITY PLAYBOOK

THE JOHN HENRY HEALTH EQUITY PLAYBOOK

A FOUR-YEAR HEALTH POLICY AGENDA FOR BLACK MEN

DR. OKEY K. ENYIA

Stay Connected to the Movement

The *John Henry Health Equity Playbook* is more than a book—it's the start and continuation of a national conversation. We want you to be part of it.

⊞ **Scan the QR code below** to visit the *official Playbook page* on my website. There you will find:

- Policy and Advocacy Consulting
- Updates and bonus resources
- Speaking and event information
- Newsletter sign-up to stay informed
- Easy links to purchase additional copies for your network

Or go directly to: https://enyiastrategies.com/books
Your engagement helps turn this playbook into a movement for change.

The Cover Story

The cover of *The John Henry Health Equity Playbook* is more than an image. It symbolizes the focus, resilience, and power of Black men, while capturing the tension between visibility and invisibility that has defined so much of our lived experience. The stark contrasts speak to the fierce urgency of now: the demand that Black men's health, voices, and futures be seen clearly and acted upon with purpose. Just as John Henry's story embodies strength and sacrifice, this cover reminds us that our identity and survival are not negotiable—they are central to the fight for equity, dignity, and justice.

Contents

Acknowledgments   11

Executive Summary   13

How to Read, Use, and Maximize this Playbook   17

A Call for Solidarity   21

Who Was John Henry?   25

The Socio-political Context   28

Relevant Frameworks   32

Pillar One   38
Physical and Mental Health as Social Drivers of Health   39

Pillar Two   58
Housing, Education, Broadband Access, and Economic Stability as
Social Drivers of Health   59

Digital Access and Broadband Infrastructure   69

Pillar Three   82
Civic Engagement, Violence Prevention, and Fatherhood Support as
Social Drivers of Health   83

Fatherhood: Supporting Black Men as Fathers   101

Conclusion   107

Four-year Plan   115

Appendix   129

A Very Practical Approach   157

Sample Call Script   161

How to Advocate for Bills   163

Additional Resources   165

Starting with Small Wins   167

Playbook Launch Campaign Prayer   169

Author Bio – Dr. Okey K. Enyia   173

Acknowledgments

First and foremost, I give all glory and honor to my Lord and Savior, Jesus Christ. This book would not exist without His divine guidance, grace, and the vision He placed on my heart. Every word reflects His calling and purpose over my life.

To my wife, Meghan Brown-Enyia, and our son, Ikenna Kelechi Enyia—thank you for your indomitable support and joy. Your love, encouragement, and patience made this journey possible.

To my parents, Dr. Samuel and Irene Enyia, your example of faith, discipline, and integrity shaped the man I have become. Your sacrifices and prayers continue to fuel my work.

To my late mother-in-law, Jeannette Marie Brown—who transitioned on Sunday, July 13, 2025, at 6:30 a.m. EST—writing this book as you transitioned was a sacred experience—one marked by reflection, reverence, and deep love. Your wisdom, grace, and unwavering belief in us were a quiet anchor during the storm. This work is a tribute to you.

To my five brilliant siblings—The Enyia League—thank you for being my lifelong circle of comradery, loyalty, and laughter. Our bond has been a constant reminder that I never walk alone.

To my extended family—thank you for your prayers, support, and belief in me even from afar. You are an essential part of my story.

To my brothers of Alpha Phi Alpha Fraternity, Inc., thank you for exemplifying scholarship, leadership, and service. Your brotherhood has nurtured and sharpened me in ways that words cannot fully capture.

To a few of the many mentors, coaches, and advisors who have poured into me over the years—Dr. Yashika Watkins, Dr. Dharius Daniels, Dr. Derek Griffith, Dr. Karriem Watson, Dr. Matthew Stevenson III, and Dr. Eugene Migliaccio—thank you for challenging me to lead with both conviction and compassion. Each of you has helped me grow not just as a professional, but as a man of purpose.

I literally would not be the man I am today without the love, support, and encouragement of all of you—and so many others whose names are not listed here but are deeply etched in my heart. This book stands as a collective offering of your investment in me.

Thank you.

Executive Summary

The **John Henry Health Equity Playbook** outlines a bold, forward-thinking four-year agenda designed to advance health equity for Black men across the United States and abroad. Named after the legendary figure John Henry, this playbook addresses the systemic challenges and unique health inequities Black men face, incorporating a structured, phased approach under three primary pillars: physical and mental health, economic stability, and community empowerment through civic engagement.

Utilizing the Social Drivers of Health (SDOH) framework, the agenda integrates existing knowledge on social, political, and economic drivers of health disparities, with a specific focus on how these factors impact Black men's health outcomes. To be clear, the social drivers of health are "the conditions in the environments where people are born, live, learn, work, play, worship, and age that affect a wide range of health, functioning, and quality-of-life outcomes and risks."[1]

Nevertheless, achieving these goals demands more than strategic planning; it requires investment. As outlined in the accompanying Investment Prospectus, eliminating racial health disparities could save the U.S. economy over $421 billion annually, with education-related health gaps costing an additional $940 billion[2]. Black men's health dis-

---

1   Social Needs and Social Determinants: The Role of the Centers for Disease Control and Prevention and Public Health
2   NIH-funded study highlights the financial toll of health disparities in the United States

parities alone contribute an estimated $31 billion per year in direct medical costs and nearly $450 billion in lost productivity and premature deaths over just three years[3].

This playbook also aligns with the *Healthy People* 2030 initiative[4], focusing on achieving health equity by addressing social drivers of health and reducing inequities experienced by Black men. *Healthy People* 2030 is a national framework developed by the U.S. Department of Health and Human Services (HHS) to guide efforts in improving the health and well-being of all Americans. Originating in 1979 with the Surgeon General's report *Healthy People: The Surgeon General's Report on Health Promotion and Disease Prevention*, it has evolved to address emerging public health challenges every decade.

To translate this vision into actionable change, the playbook is organized around three interconnected pillars that serve as the foundation for a healthier, more equitable future for Black men. Each pillar is rooted in evidence, policy, and practice—deliberately designed to confront the structural forces that shape health outcomes. Together, these pillars reflect a comprehensive strategy that not only addresses immediate health needs but also invests in long-term solutions—across healthcare, economic opportunity, and civic life—that uplift individuals, families, and entire communities. Below is an at-a-glance overview of each pillar and its role in advancing this agenda.

The Three Pillars At-a-glance

Pillar One focuses on enhancing healthcare infrastructure and access. This pillar includes policies aimed at eliminating healthcare inequities by promoting culturally humble care, increasing representation of Black men in healthcare professions, expanding mental health and substance use disorder services, and advocating for affordable health insurance options.

---

3   The Economic Burden of Health Inequalities in the United States
4   *Healthy People 2030*

Pillar Two focuses on housing, education, broadband access, and economic stability—essential building blocks for health and long-term prosperity. By advancing homeownership, expanding educational pathways, boosting job training, and closing wage gaps, this pillar targets the roots of economic inequities. Community-based organizations are vital partners in driving these solutions forward. The stakes are high: racial and ethnic health disparities already cost over $421 billion from the U.S. economy each year with education-related gaps costing an additional $940 billion[5].

Men's health disparities, especially among Black men, fuel these losses; however, targeted investment can reverse the trend. Noted earlier, Black men's health disparities cost the U.S. economy over $31 billion annually in direct medical expenses and nearly $450 billion over three years when factoring in lost productivity and premature death[6]. Closing these gaps is both a moral and economic imperative to strengthen communities, reduce healthcare costs, and drive national prosperity.

Pillar Three champions civic engagement, violence prevention, and fatherhood support. Civic engagement is framed as a crucial determinant of health, fostering healthier communities by empowering Black men to influence policies that shape their lives. This pillar also tackles violence prevention through community-based interventions, trauma-informed care, and economic support. Lastly, it recognizes the importance of supporting Black fathers in fostering family stability and child well-being, providing policy recommendations for fatherhood engagement, economic stability, and mental health support.

This playbook advances a vision rooted in health equity, policy innovation, and community empowerment. It takes a bipartisan, bicameral approach—recognizing that the health and well-being of Black men is not a partisan issue, but a shared national imperative should be addressed across the entire political spectrum.

---

5   Study shows steep financial costs of healthcare inequities

6   Health Disparities Among African-American and Hispanic Men Cost Economy More Than $450B Over Four Years

How to Read, Use, and Maximize this Playbook

The *John Henry Health Equity Playbook* is more than a policy document—it is a movement-building tool. Whether you are a policymaker, advocate, practitioner, entrepreneur, or concerned citizen, this guide is designed to help you turn insight into action and build a healthier, more equitable future for Black men and the broader community. Here is how to get the most out of it:

1. **Read with Intention**

   a) Learn from John Henry's story as a powerful metaphor for the resilience, labor, and health burden Black men carry.
   b) Dive into each pillar (health, economic stability, and civic engagement) with an eye toward what is most relevant to your work or community.

2. **Use it as a Strategic Toolkit**

   a) Each section includes data, recommendations, and proposed policy solutions. Use these (please cite this playbook as a source) as a foundation for grant proposals, legislative advocacy, community planning, or public testimony.

b) The Policy Advocacy Framework in the appendix offers step-by-step guidance on lobbying, organizing, and stakeholder engagement.

3. **Collaborate Across Sectors**

a) The Playbook is intentionally multidisciplinary. Whether you work in public health, education, housing, justice reform, artificial intelligence/machine learning, or fatherhood programs, you will find actionable guidance that invites collaboration.
b) Form coalitions with community-based organizations, fraternities, sororities, faith leaders, researchers, and government allies to co-create solutions.

4. **Take a Four-Year Approach**

a) Follow the year-by-year roadmap to implement change across short-, medium, and long-term horizons.
b) Use the First 100 Days, Midterm Strategy, and Fatherhood/Family Initiatives to plan programming and advocacy campaigns over time.

5. **Measure What Matters**

a) Reference the metrics provided in each section to track your progress and evaluate outcomes.
b) Leverage the frameworks in the appendix (e.g., Targeted Universalism, Political Determinants of Health) to shape equitable, scalable policies.

6. **Center Black Men's Voices**

a) The Playbook is grounded in African American Male Theory (AAMT), which insists that Black men are not problems to be solved—but assets to be invested in.

b) Use this lens to guide how you design programs, fund initiatives, and tell stories.

7. **Engage, Share, and Activate**

   a) Share insights from the playbook in meetings, presentations, town halls, and digital campaigns.
   b) Use the content to train others, empower youth, and spark conversations about systemic change.
   c) Invite others to join the movement by downloading the playbook, supporting aligned legislation, or participating in Men's Health Month each June.

Pro Tip: This Playbook is a living document. Mark it up. Highlight what speaks to you. Bring it to your meetings. Share excerpts in grant applications and strategy decks. Let it be your guide and your blueprint.

An Additional Note to the Reader:

Throughout this playbook, you will encounter short, fictionalized vignettes that introduce specific sections. These stories follow a character named **John Henry**—a modern embodiment of the legendary figure whose strength, sacrifice, and resilience mirror the real lives of so many Black men today.

These narrative moments are designed to center lived experience, evoke emotion, and humanize the data and policy recommendations that follow. While fictional, they are drawn from a composite of truths—shaped by research, historical context, and personal reflection, including insights from my own life story as shared in *Indisputable: The Story of a Favored Son* that you can find on my website https://enyiastrategies.com/.

By including these vignettes, I aim to remind every reader that this playbook is not just about policy. It is about people. It is about you—because this is where purpose meets policy.

A Call for Solidarity

"When it comes to the health of children, it is a woman's health and well-being that is paramount and most important. When it comes to the health of the family and community, it is the man's health and well-being that is paramount and most important."
-Ambrose Lane Jr.

Black men are not a monolith. Our lives are shaped by intersecting identities, including class, sexuality, immigration status, ability, geography, and more. There is power in solidarity; and partnership produces progress. To be clear, we are not advocating for men's health at the expense of women's health. Rather, we believe that by working in solidarity with families and loved ones, we can build healthier communities.

Moreover, health equity is not a zero-sum game. Efforts to advance the well-being of Black men do not diminish the importance of family, gender equity, or community health. Instead, they are a vital and overdue complement. True equity uplifts everyone by recognizing and addressing the unique needs of all populations, including men.

Best-selling author, Heather McGee, takes a similar stance in the context of the impacts of racism across ecosystems[7]. Just as decades of investment in women's health have yielded transformative benefits for families and society, a focused commitment to Black men's health can strengthen entire communities. Men's health equity is family health equity. When our fathers, brothers, partners, and sons are well—physically, mentally, and emotionally—our families are stronger, our communities are more resilient, and our public health systems are more effective.

Therefore, this playbook emphasizes strategic advocacy at all levels of government, aligning with recent policy initiatives to create systemic, long-term change. By following the guidance laid out in this playbook, policymakers, community organizations, and advocates—bringing people together from all walks of life—can collaboratively dismantle systemic barriers and improve the health, stability, and socioeconomic conditions for Black men, their families, and their communities.

The Four-Year Strategic Roadmap

This playbook outlines a phased, four-year strategy informed by interviews, focus groups, meetings, summits, conferences, and conventions:

- **Year 1:** Build critical infrastructure by launching targeted health, housing, education, and economic initiatives.
- **Year 2:** Institutionalize systems change and embed civic engagement as a health equity tool.
- **Year 3:** Strengthen families and leadership pipelines by advancing fatherhood programs and securing long-term sustainability.
- **Year 4:** Sustain and scale progress by expanding local and state adoption and rigorously evaluating impact.

---

7   The Sum of Us: What Racism Costs Everyone and How We Can Prosper Together

Each phase builds upon the last, ensuring that health equity for Black men becomes embedded, enduring, and transformative. To ground this health equity agenda in both historical symbolism and contemporary urgency, we turn to the story of John Henry—a powerful figure whose legacy embodies the resilience, challenges, and aspirations at the heart of this work.

Who Was John Henry?

The legend of John Henry[8] tells the story of an exceptionally strong and skilled Black railroad worker in the late 19th century. He was known for his work as a steel-driver, hammering steel spikes into rocks to make way for railroad tunnels. In a famous contest against a steam-powered drill, John Henry outperformed the machine by drilling deeper but tragically died from exhaustion immediately after his victory.

While John Henry has long been understood as a folkloric figure, historical research suggests he was also a real person whose life was shaped by the brutal system of post-Civil War racial control. According to historian Scott Reynolds Nelson, John Henry was a nineteen-year-old Black man from New Jersey who was convicted of theft in a Virginia court in 1866 and sentenced to ten years of hard labor[9].

Rather than serving his sentence in a traditional prison, Henry was forced into the convict-leasing system, a state-sanctioned practice

---

8   The John Henryism Hypothesis
9   Steel Drivin' Man: John Henry, the Untold Story of an American Legend

that supplied incarcerated Black men as cheap, expendable labor to private industries. He was leased to work on the construction of the Chesapeake & Ohio (C&O) Railroad, where incarcerated men labored under extreme and deadly conditions alongside emerging steam-powered drills. At the Lewis Tunnel site in West Virginia, the convergence of human bodies and industrial machinery symbolized a broader historical moment: the transformation of Black freedom into coerced labor through law, punishment, and economic exploitation.

This historical context frames John Henry as an important symbol in the field of Black men's health[10] because his story reflects themes of physical strength, endurance, and the burden of labor, often at the cost of personal health and well-being. His story also highlights the broader socio-political and economic conditions that affect Black men's health, such as the systemic exploitation of labor[11], racial disparities and inequities in healthcare[12], and the neglect of mental and physical well-being in the face of societal pressures[13].

In a more contemporary context, the author of the "John Henryism Hypothesis," Dr. Sherman James served as a catalyst for better understanding the connections between the need to 'work harder' and its implications for chronic health conditions like heart disease in Black Americans[14]. Dr. James grounded his scholarship in lived experience through *The Narrative of John Henry Martin*, based on his 1978 interview with John Henry Martin. Born in 1907, John Henry Martin was a retired North Carolina farmer who ultimately succeeded in freeing his family from debt, though at significant cost to his health[15].

---

10   Racial Discrimination, John Henryism, and Depression Among African Americans
11   Discrimination, Harassment, Abuse and Bullying in the Workplace: Contribution of Workplace Injustice to Occupational Health Disparities
12   Men's Health Equity: A Handbook
13   Visible and Invisible Trends in Black Men's Health: Pitfalls and Promises for Addressing Racial, Ethnic, and Gender Inequities in Health
14   John Henryism and the Health of African-Americans
15   The Narrative of John Henry Martin

More recently, an article[16] examined how COVID-19 disproportion-ately impacted young Black men in the U.S., linking severe health and economic effects to the John Henryism Hypothesis. Failing to address the health and well-being of Black men carries significant socio-political consequences, impacting everything from economic stability and healthcare costs to community trust and civic engagement.

---

16   How COVID-19 Hollowed Out a Generation of Young Black Men

The Socio-political Context

In October 2024, the Harris-Walz presidential campaign committed to creating an Opportunity Economy where everyone has the chance not just to survive, but to thrive. Former Vice President Kamala Harris used her platform to acknowledge that Black men[17] have often felt their voices are overlooked in the political process; and that there is immense untapped ambition and leadership within the Black male community. Black men and boys deserve transformational leadership who will unlock their talent and potential by dismantling historical barriers to wealth creation, education, employment, earnings, health, and by reforming the criminal justice system.

Consequently, we remain undeterred in our resolve to advocate for our health and well-being. Dean of Global Health and Meharry Medical College, Daniel Dawes, stated "The movement to advance health equity for all in our nation does not stop based on an election." To his point, if you are not at the decision-making table, you are on the menu—and all "politics" is local. This Playbook is one approach to ensuring that Black men have a seat at every decision-making table; and not just to have a seat, but also to serve as a credible voice. The strength of a democracy lies in each generation's commitment to protect it, and this playbook aims to provide a framework for finding common ground across Republican Sand Democrat administrations. To be clear, as we

---

17   Opportunity Agenda for Black Men

navigate an increasingly polarized political landscape, *The John Henry Health Equity Playbook* is deliberately structured to transcend party lines and legislative chambers. In a government shaped by diverse political affiliations, it reflects a commitment to working across party lines and across chambers to enact policies that elevate Black men as a foundation for stronger, more equitable communities.

Policy Neglect

Noted author, Damon Young stated, "It's hard to fight for your health when you're fighting for your humanity." The concept of Black male "invisibility" is metaphorically explored in Ralph Ellison's *Invisible Man* (1952), which describes a nameless Black man's journey during the Great Migration. His experiences reflect how socio-political power structures perpetuate negative stereotypes such as criminality and ineptitude, marginalizing him and the broader Black male population. Despite being hyper-visible in the criminal justice system, Black men are largely invisible in research and policies aimed at improving their health and well-being.

This policy neglect is exacerbated by a lack of political will, as those in power often exclude marginalized communities from research and legislative agendas, hindering meaningful change[18]. We must connect the dots between the nuances of the policy-making process and the lived realities of Black men every day. For example, studies[19] have found that voting up and down the ballot (i.e., local, state, and federal levels) is intrinsically linked to people's health and well-being. In other words, a civically engaged community is a healthy community.

This agenda is intentionally designed to be resilient across political transitions. While it centers the lived experiences of Black men, it reflects American values: family, fairness, faith, freedom, and economic opportunity. Investing in Black men's health uplifts working

---

18   The Social Construction of Target Populations
19   Voter Participation Is a Path to Health Equity: How Health Departments Can Promote a Healthy, Inclusive Democracy

families, enhances public safety, and reduces long-term healthcare costs. These are bipartisan concerns—and this playbook provides a blueprint for addressing them across ideological lines.

As Black Men: What Do We Want and What Do We Believe?

Black men represent diverse subgroups with distinct cultural, socio-economic, and immigration backgrounds, including American-born Black men, Caribbean Black men, and African immigrants. Research has shown critical differences among these groups in health care access and utilization, such as health insurance being positively associated with having a usual source of care for American-born Black men but negatively associated among Caribbean Black men[20]. Additionally, studies have highlighted the compounded impact of intersecting structural oppressions on the health of Black sexual minority men, emphasizing the need for intersectional approaches in health research and interventions[21]. Moreover, the relationship chronic conditions, aging, and disability among the Black male population indicates that chronic health issues disproportionately affect this community, necessitating targeted public health strategies[22].

Oppressive social and governance structures are most comfortable when we remain silent. As Black men we want to be intentionally and sustainably prioritized on policy and research agendas[23]—ensuring equitable access to quality healthcare[24], equitable health insurance coverage[25], the dismantling of structural racism in healthcare[26], community-based health interventions[27], comprehensive education on

---

20   Determinants of Usual Source of Care Disparities Among African American and Caribbean Black Men: Findings from the National Survey of American Life
21   Intersecting Structural Oppression and Black Sexual Minority Men's Health
22   Relationship Between Chronic Conditions and Disability in African American Men and Women
23   Examining the Affordable Care Act and its Impact on Access to Care for Black Men and White Men: Implications for Policy and Practice
24   Usual Source of Care and Access to Care in the US: 2005 v. 2015
25   Health Coverage by Race and Ethnicity, 2010-2022
26   Structural Racism and Health Inequities in the USA: Evidence and Interventions
27   Community Needs and Recommendations for Multilevel Mental Health Interventions Among Young Black Men with Previous Trauma Exposure

Black men's health[28], increased representation of Black men in allied health professions[29], targeted research on Black men's physical and mental health[30], economic empowerment[31], environmental justice[32], and a holistic approach to health and wellness[33]—because we believe that these are essential for achieving health equity, addressing racial disparities, and improving health outcomes for Black men.

The Call to Action

Our call to action is shaped by African American Male Theory (AAMT)[34]. This theory provides a unique perspective on the experiences of Black men, addressing systemic racism, socio-political challenges, and identity issues that traditional frameworks often overlook. Incorporating AAMT reinforces the policy agenda's commitment to centering Black men's lived experiences in health equity-related policies. This framework is particularly relevant in shaping policies that address the invisibility of Black men in healthcare, educational opportunities, and socio-economic development. By aligning AAMT with this agenda, we promote an evidence-based approach that targets the root causes of inequities and advocates for transformative structural change.

We must proceed with a long-game strategy that incorporates short-term tactics to ensure we can capitalize on policy windows. To be clear, this is a fluid, yet strategic four-year roadmap that can be tailored to unique needs, interests, and timelines. The next section will describe relevant frameworks that can help shape policy and practice for Black men. Likewise, a high-level outline of how the Opportunity Agenda for Black Men mapped to the social drivers of health can be found in the appendix.

---

28   Men's Health Equity: A Handbook
29   Black men make up less than 3% of physicians, which requires immediate action, say leaders in academic medicine.
30   "Centering the Margins": Moving Equity to the Center of Men's Health Research
31   Black Men and the U.S. Economy: How the Economic Recovery Is Perpetuating Systemic Racism
32   Environmental Justice Radar: A Tool for Community-Based Mapping to Increase Environmental Awareness and Participatory Decision Making
33   Black Male Initiative Launches today
34   Introducing African American Male Theory

Relevant Frameworks

The following frameworks align with examining and *operationalizing* ways in which the health and well-being of historically marginalized communities like Black men can be accounted for in terms of policy and practice. More details can be found in the appendix.

- "The Political Determinants of Health," Daniel Dawes provides a framework[35] for conceptualizing the ways in which policy decisions impact every facet of our lives.

- To help "operationalize" historically marginalized voices, the Commonwealth Fund developed a framework[36], "Engaging the Voice to Support Racially Equitable Policymaking," that focuses on involving historically marginalized communities in policy-making to advance racial equity.

- An intersectional approach[37] not only helps explain which social characteristics impact health but *why* those factors impact health. However, a bio-psycho-social approach accounts for not only the range of factors that determine risk but the range

---

35   The Political Determinants of Health
36   Engaging Voice to Support Racially Equitable Decision-making
37   An Intersectional Approach to Men's Health

of places that targeted interventions may be most impactful for Black men[38].

- The Centers for Disease Control and Prevention (CDC) framework[39] for addressing Social Determinants of Health (SDOH) emphasizes the vital role of non-medical factors in health outcomes and advocates for a proactive approach to improve population health and advance health equity.

- Professor Ruqaiijah Yearby proposed a revised SDOH framework[40] that emphasizes structural and systemic drivers of health inequities, specifically how social, economic, and political forces shape health outcomes across populations. It expands traditional SDOH concepts by focusing on root causes, such as institutionalized discrimination and historical injustices, that systematically disadvantage marginalized groups. This framework suggests actionable pathways, including policy reform, community engagement, and advocacy efforts, to dismantle inequities by addressing upstream determinants like housing, education, and employment conditions, all while incorporating health justice principles.

- The National Institutes of Minority and Health Disparities Research Framework[41] is a comprehensive model that highlights diverse health determinants critical to understanding and addressing minority health and health disparities. This framework helps to evaluate progress, identify gaps, and uncover opportunities within the NIMHD and NIH research portfolios focused on these areas. The model emphasizes that health outcomes are influenced by multiple levels and includes a life course perspective, underscoring the significance of

---

38 Examining the Affordable Care Act and its Impact on Access to Care for Black Men and White Men: Implications for Policy and Practice
39 Centers for Disease Control and Prevention Social Determinants of Health Framework
40 Structural Racism and Health Disparities: Reconfiguring the Social Determinants of Health Framework to Include the Root Cause
41 NIMHD Minority Health and Health Disparities Research Framework

examining factors across an individual's lifespan to understand health disparities. The framework's factors are illustrative rather than exhaustive, and its focus on specific populations and elements may evolve over time.

- The Targeted Universalism framework[42], developed by Dr. John A. Powell at UC Berkeley's Othering & Belonging Institute, is an approach to achieving social equity that combines universal goals with targeted strategies for specific groups. It acknowledges that different populations may require unique interventions to overcome varied barriers and reach the same universal goal. Supporting Black men is not an exclusionary act—it is a strategic investment in the health, stability, and prosperity of our entire nation. Research[43] shows that when we reduce disparities for the most marginalized, we uplift all communities through stronger economies, safer neighborhoods, and more resilient families. Just as the curb-cut effect[44] in disability policy created benefits for delivery workers and parents with strollers, targeted policies that empower Black men can create widespread societal gains. This is the essence of Targeted Universalism: advancing universal goals through tailored strategies.

- *Healthy People* 2030 outlines 355 measurable objectives across diverse topics, such as chronic disease prevention, mental health, maternal and child health, and access to care. These objectives serve as benchmarks for federal, state, and local stakeholders to guide policies, programs, and funding. The initiative emphasizes cross-sector collaboration, evidence-based practices, and tracking progress using reliable data systems like the National Health Interview Survey (NHIS). While progress is ongoing, *Healthy People* 2030 aims to adapt to changing

---

42   Targeted Universalism
43   Targeted Universalism Case Studies
44   The Curb-Cut Effect and the Perils of Accessibility without Disability

public health needs, ensuring it remains relevant and impactful in addressing the nation's health challenges.

- Too often, discussions surrounding Black men's health focus on disparities, risks, and deficits—painting a picture of vulnerability rather than resilience. While addressing inequities is necessary, it is equally important to highlight the assets, leadership, and innovations that Black men bring to every sector of society, particularly in the realm of health. The BMe Community asset-framing model[45] takes a strengths-based approach and shifts the focus from what Black men lack to what they contribute: as healthcare professionals, caregivers, mentors, community leaders, entrepreneurs, policy influencers, and changemakers. More detailed information on a strengths-based or asset-based approach in the context of Black men can be found in the appendix.

These frameworks collectively address health equity by highlighting how policies, non-medical factors, and structural forces influence health outcomes. Likewise, it is recognized that technology can be a critical tool to meet Black men where they are— bridging access gaps, enhancing service delivery, supporting education, building economic opportunity, expanding civic engagement, and preventing violence. Technology must be deployed thoughtfully to ensure cultural relevance, to protect privacy, and to address the digital divide. Therefore, we also intentionally integrate ways in which technology can serve as a catalyst for advancing health equity for Black men. The next section will describe the three foundational pillars referenced earlier.

---

45   Asset-framing

A John Henry Story: "The Waiting Room"

John Henry sat waiting in the corner of an emergency room lobby, his shoulders hunched under the weight of more than just chest pain. He had felt the tightness for three days now—an ache that pulsed from his sternum to his back like a slow-burning fuse. But like most men he knew, he had worked through it. Worked past it.

He had promised his daughter he would be at her school play, and he had already missed too much. No paid sick days. No nearby urgent care. And besides, he did not trust hospitals—not after what happened to his uncle who went in for a routine check-up and never came back.

When the nurse finally called his name, John Henry stood slowly. No one had told him the signs of a silent heart attack. No one had checked on him since he left his factory job five months ago. No doctor had ever asked about his diet, his sleep, his stress.

Inside the exam room, he noticed the pamphlets on the wall—none showed faces like his. The young resident barely made eye contact. The machines beeped. The fluorescent lights buzzed.

John Henry was more than a patient. He was a living ledger of structural neglect. A Black man whose chart read "elevated risk," but whose life had never been treated like a priority.

He did not want pity. He wanted answers.

He wanted care. He wanted to live.

Physical and Mental Health as Social Drivers of Health

"We can't heal what we won't face." **- Ta-Nehisi Coates**

Pillar one presents data and outlines strategies to address the systemic barriers that contribute to significant health disparities among Black men, focusing on improving chronic and mental health outcomes through policies that expand healthcare access, enhance education, foster community support, increase workforce diversity, and empower community-based organizations to implement targeted interventions.

Physical Health

Black men experience poor health outcomes across a spectrum of chronic medical conditions and comorbidities (e.g., cardiovascular disease, cancer, obesity, diabetes, etc.) that ultimately lead to lower quality of life and premature death[46]:

- As of 2022, the average life expectancy for Black men in the United States was 72.8 years compared to 77.5 years for white

---

46   Why Black Men in America Have Worse Health than White Men–and What Needs to Change

men[47]. This has been an entrenched gap for decades. A 2009 study by former U.S. Surgeon General Dr. David Satcher found that the mortality rate for Black men ages 45 to 54 was more than twice the rate for white men in the same age group[48].

- Another study found that the mortality rate for young Black men (ages 20-24) is staggeringly high at 61 per 100,000 population, compared to 5.1 per 100,000 for white men of the same age group[49].

- The literature is replete with studies showing that bias and fear of Black men likely result in them not getting the same healthcare as white male patients[50].

- Long-standing disparities and inequities that negatively impact Black men can be mapped, in part, to the lack of sustainable, robust, and targeted research funding awards for researchers who desire to support Black men and their health[51].

- Studies have found that Black principal investigators were significantly underrepresented even after adjusting for career stage and degrees, with Black principal investigators being 40% less likely than their White colleagues to be a principal investigator[52].

- Black men make up less than 3% of all physicians in the United States and the number of Black men enrolled in medical school has decreased between 1978 and 2014[53].

- The Tuskegee Syphilis Experiment (1932-1972) was an unethical study conducted by the U.S. Public Health Service on Black

---

47 Key Data on Health and Health Care by Race and Ethnicity
48 What If We Were Equal? A Comparison of the Black-White Mortality Gap in 1960 and 2000
49 Vital Signs: Racial Disparities in Age-specific Mortality Among Blacks or African Americans—United States, 1999-2015
50 Healthcare Providers' Formative Experiences with Race and Black Male Patients in Urban Hospital Environment
51 Race, Ethnicity, and NIH Research Awards
52 Racial Inequity in Grant Funding from the US National Institutes of Health
53 Black men make up less than 3% of physicians. That requires immediate action, say leaders in academic medicine.

men in Macon County, Alabama. Researchers deliberately withheld treatment for syphilis from participants, even after penicillin became the standard cure in 1947. The experiment not only eroded trust but also highlighted the systemic failure of institutions to be trustworthy by reinforcing the need for transparency, ethical research, and accountability in healthcare to rebuild confidence in medical institutions.

- At the same time, Black men are significantly underrepresented in clinical trials. For instance, a study focusing on oncology clinical trials found that Black men comprised less than 5% of the participants[54].

- Black men are significantly underrepresented in the physician assistant and associate (PA) profession compared to their share of the United States population. The share of Black men who matriculated into PA programs averaged 1.2 percent from 2012 to 2021 (less than Black men's 8.7 percent share of the United States population for individuals aged 20 to 29)[55].

- Black men are less likely to visit the dentist, are twice as likely to experience tooth decay, and have a significantly lower five-year oral cancer survival rate when compared to White men[56].

- One study found that structural racism and anti-LGBTQIA policies were associated with worse health outcomes among Black gay, bisexual, and other sexual minority men (SMM), highlighting the compounding impact of intersecting oppressions on their health[57].

- Black men in the U.S. have the highest lifetime risk of developing kidney failure. In 2018, they accounted for 16.6% of all

54   Racial and Ethnic Representation of Participants in US Clinical Trials of New Drugs and Biologics
55   Black Men Remain Underrepresented in the Physician Assistant Profession
56   Assessing the Oral Health Needs of African American Men in Low-income, Urban Communities
57   Intersecting Structural Oppression and Black Sexual Minority Men's Health

kidney failure patients, despite representing just 6.4% of the total U.S. population[58].

- Black men often reside in neighborhoods with limited access to quality healthcare, nutritious food, and safe recreational spaces. These areas may also have higher exposure to environmental pollutants, contributing to chronic health issues[59].

Just as John Henry's body bore the weight of physical exhaustion, so too did his mind carry invisible wounds. For Black men across the country, the struggle for health is not only physical—it is psychological, emotional, and spiritual. The next section turns our attention to the often-unseen crisis: mental health and substance use.

A John Henry Story: "The Barbershop Smile"

You would never guess anything was wrong by the way John Henry laughed in the barbershop. Loud. Quick. Charismatic. That smile—sharp as a straight razor—was his shield.

What folks did not see was the silence that swallowed him whole once he got home. The nights he sat in the dark, staring at the same bottle he swore he would not touch. The texts he started to send asking for help—but never finished. After all, real men did not ask for help.

Especially not Black men.

Especially not him.

He had grown up hearing phrases like "man up" and "pray it away." Therapy was for other people—rich people, white people. Not for someone like him, someone who worked two jobs, sent money to his mom, and still could not sleep more than four hours without waking up in a cold sweat.

---

58   Lifetime Incidence of CKD Stages 3-5 in the United States
59   Visible and Invisible Trends in Black Men's Health: Pitfalls and Promises for Addressing Racial, Ethnic, and Gender Inequities in Health

The one time he tried calling a local clinic, he was told the next available appointment was six weeks out. When he showed up, the intake form asked questions that did not make sense. The receptionist did not look him in the eye. This time, he hung up before giving his name.

John Henry did not need a lecture. He needed someone who looked like him, who understood why crying in public could get you labeled, why being vulnerable could be dangerous, and why every day felt like survival.

He wasn't weak. He was tired. He wasn't broken. He was ignored. And he wasn't alone—but he sure felt like it.

Mental Health and Substance Use as Social Drivers of Health

Regarding mental health, one reason Black men might hesitate to discuss their mental health challenges is the stigma attached to mental health within the Black community. Traditionally, mental illness has often been perceived as a weakness or a lack of faith, which has led many Black men to feel shame or embarrassment when considering seeking help for these issues[60].

However, structural barriers play a very significant role in perpetuating the lack of culturally-humble mental health professionals and a lack of targeted, sustained support for Black men in the substance use disorder ecosystem. This section presents data on the mental health challenges Black men face, highlighting the impact of stigma, the shortage of culturally humble providers, and systemic barriers that limit access to effective mental health and substance use disorder treatment—underscoring the need for targeted, accessible support within underserved communities.

- According to the American Psychological Association in 2015, "86 percent of psychologists in the U.S. workforce were white,

---

60   Why Black Men Don't Open Up: Mental Health Stigma in the Black Community

5 percent were Asian, 5 percent were Hispanic, 4 percent were Black/African-American and 1 percent were multiracial or from other racial/ethnic groups[61]."

- Children and adolescents in racial, ethnic, sexual, gender and other minority groups experience inequities in access to care and disparities in outcomes for mental and behavioral health conditions. Suicide rates are nearly twice as high for Black boys compared to White boys 5–11 years old and have been increasing disproportionately among adolescent Black girls 12–17 years old[62].

- Another study highlighted disparities in substance use treatment access for racial and ethnic minorities, specifically examining how community factors influence the timely receipt of services among Black, American Indian, Latino, and White clients in Washington State. For Black men, the findings revealed that they are less likely to initiate or engage in treatment compared to white clients, even when community factors such as economic disadvantage and racial composition are considered. This delay in receiving treatment contributes to prolonged substance use challenges and potentially worsens related health outcomes for Black men, emphasizing the need for targeted policies to improve access and address barriers within under-resourced communities[63].

State of Cannabis Policy in the Context of Black Men and Boys

Cannabis policy in the U.S. remains a patchwork of state-level legalization efforts against the backdrop of federal prohibition. Despite increasing public support, with 88% of Americans favoring some form of legalization, cannabis remains a Schedule I drug under federal law, impeding research and creating legal uncertainties.[64] While 38 states and Washington, D.C., allow medical marijuana, 24 states permit recreational use, and several others have decriminalized possession.

The health benefits of marijuana include pain relief, appetite stimulation, and symptom management for conditions such as multiple sclerosis, HIV/AIDS, and chemotherapy-induced nausea.[65] However, marijuana use also presents risks such as memory impairment, lung damage, increased addiction potential, and impaired driving ability.[66] Emerging research indicates that early cannabis use alters brain structure, potentially increasing the risk for substance use disorder later in life, particularly among adolescents from historically marginalized communities.[67] Another study suggested that chronic cannabis use could lead to an increased risk of heart disease[68]. The lack of rigorous federal research and clinical trials due to marijuana's classification remains a barrier to fully understanding its medical potential and long-term health effects. This is not about choosing sides on cannabis use; it is about bringing overdue attention to a complex issue with far-reaching implications. Stakeholders across public health, education, policy, and community sectors must be engaged in a more intentional and informed dialogue.

For Black men and boys, cannabis policy is not just a health issue—it is a social justice issue deeply intertwined with the war on drugs, racialized criminalization, and economic disparities. Decades of disproportionate policing and incarceration for marijuana-related offenses have devastated Black communities, yet Black entrepreneurs remain largely excluded from the legal cannabis industry due to high licensing fees, capital access barriers, and state-mandated compliance costs.[69]

---

64   Most Americans Favor Legalizing Marijuana for Medical, Recreational Use
65   Therapeutic Effects of Cannabis and Cannabinoids
66   Adverse Health Effects of Marijuana Use
67   Cannabis and Teens
68   Marijuana Smoking and THC-Edible Use
69   Road to 2030: Federal Legislative Solutions to Social Equity in a Booming Cannabis Industry

Additionally, despite marijuana decriminalization and legalization in many states, racial disparities in cannabis-related arrests persist, highlighting the need for further policy reform. Moreover, Black men face greater barriers to addiction treatment and mental health care, making harm reduction strategies crucial.[70] Current research underscores the need for culturally responsive prevention programs targeting Black youth, particularly given the increasing evidence that cannabis use affects brain development and cognition.[71] Expanding economic opportunities within the legal cannabis market while simultaneously addressing public health risks is essential to ensuring equitable cannabis policy.

Advancing cannabis policy requires a bipartisan, bicameral approach to ensure durable, equitable reform. With champions on both sides of the aisle and in both chambers—like Representatives Dina Titus and Brian Mast; and Senators Cory Booker and Rand Paul—real progress depends on cross-party, cross-chamber collaboration. This approach increases the chance of enacting comprehensive legislation that addresses public health, criminal justice, and economic equity, while avoiding the pitfalls of partisan gridlock and policy reversals.

Proposed Health Policy Recommendations

- **Strengthen Pathways to Health Professions:**

    o **Diverse Medical Workforce:**
      Implement targeted recruitment and retention strategies to increase the representation of Black men in medical and health-related fields. A diverse workforce can enhance cultural competence and improve health outcomes in underserved communities.

---

70   Treatment Disparities among African American Men with Depression: Implications for Clinical Practice
71   Preventing Marijuana Use Among Youth

- **Expand Health Insurance Coverage:**

  o **Medicaid Expansion:** Encourage states to expand Medicaid under the *Affordable Care Act* to cover more low-income individuals, reducing uninsured rates among Black men.

  o **Affordable Health Plans:** Increase subsidies and reduce premiums for marketplace health insurance plans to make coverage more accessible.

- **Health Literacy Programs:** Incorporate health education into school curricula to empower students with knowledge about preventive care and healthy lifestyles.

- **Community Health Initiatives:** Develop community-based programs that provide health education and resources, particularly in areas with high disparities. Hospitals can partner with educational institutions to create training curricula that equip community health workers with the necessary skills to address community-specific health challenges.

- **Address Social Drivers of Health:**

  o **Economic Opportunities:** Create job training and employment programs that offer stable, well-paying jobs with health benefits.

  o **Safe Living Environments:** Invest in community development projects that improve housing, reduce crime, and provide access to recreational facilities.

  o **Technology:** Leverage telehealth platforms to increase culturally humble healthcare access for Black men, particularly in underserved areas where physical proximity to clinics remains a barrier.

- **Implement Bias and Cultural Humility Training:**

    o **Healthcare Providers:** Mandate training for healthcare professionals to address implicit biases and improve cultural sensitivity, ensuring equitable treatment for all patients.

    o **Educational Institutions:** Provide similar training for educators to foster inclusive learning environments.

- **Enhance Data Collection and Research:**

    o **Disaggregated Data:** Collect and analyze data on health and education outcomes by race, gender, socioeconomic status and other intersectional identities to identify and address specific disparities.

    o **Community-Based Research:** Support studies that involve community members in identifying challenges and developing tailored interventions.

- **Promote Policy Advocacy and Community Engagement:**

    o **Stakeholder Collaboration (i.e., webinars, virtual town halls, social media, podcasts, etc.):** Engage community leaders, policymakers, and organizations in developing and advocating for policies that address educational and health disparities. Form coalitions with medical societies (e.g., National Medical Association, American Society of Nephrology) to submit formal comments during CMS rulemaking periods. Engage with the Medicare Payment Advisory Commission (MedPAC) to highlight disparities and propose solutions.

    o **Public Awareness Campaigns:** Launch initiatives to raise awareness about the importance of education and health equity. Engage Congressional committees overseeing CMS (e.g., House Ways & Means, Senate Finance) to introduce legislation or oversight hearings focused on health disparities, like chronic kidney disease.

Implementing these policies requires a coordinated effort among federal, state, and local governments, educational institutions, healthcare providers, and communities to create an equitable society where education and health disparities are significantly reduced.

Proposed Policy and Practice Recommendations

1. Decriminalization and Expungement of Marijuana-related Convictions

- Advocate for federal and state-level policies that decriminalize marijuana and automatically expunge prior convictions, ensuring that Black men are no longer disproportionately harmed by outdated drug laws.

- Support for collection and public reporting on cannabis-related arrests, prosecutions, and convictions, disaggregated by race.

- Provide Black men with directories of licensed medical marijuana dispensaries and programs.

- Implement retroactive sentencing reforms to address individuals currently incarcerated for nonviolent marijuana offenses.

2. Equitable Access to Medical Marijuana

- Ensure that Black men have equal access to medical marijuana programs, particularly for treating chronic conditions such as sickle cell disease, post-traumatic stress disorder (PTSD), and neuropathic pain.

- Consider collaborating with the Society of Cannabis Clinicians.

- Remove financial and bureaucratic barriers to obtaining medical marijuana cards, including insurance coverage for cannabis-based treatments.

3. Community-based Prevention and Education Programs

- Develop culturally tailored public health campaigns on the risks and benefits of marijuana, particularly addressing concerns such as cognitive impairment, bone density loss, and addiction risks.

- Direct a portion of cannabis tax revenue or other funds towards community-based programs and services in neighborhoods most impacted.

- Invest in youth-targeted interventions that educate Black boys on cannabis use's neurological and social implications, incorporating findings from NIH-supported brain imaging studies on early cannabis exposure.

4. Investment in Black-owned Cannabis Businesses

- Support Black men in creating and sustaining small businesses.

- Implement funding programs that provide Black entrepreneurs with grants, low-interest loans, and technical assistance to enter the cannabis industry.

- Mandate equity licensing programs that prioritize Black-owned businesses and reinvest cannabis tax revenues into Black communities disproportionately affected by prohibition.

5. Harm Reduction and Mental Health Support

- Expand mental health and substance use disorder treatment services for Black men, integrating cannabis use disorder treatment into existing behavioral health initiatives.

- Train healthcare providers in culturally competent addiction treatment, ensuring that Black men receive non-punitive, community-based support rather than criminalization.

6. Federal Reclassification and Research Expansion

- Advocate for removing marijuana from Schedule I classification, enabling large-scale clinical trials to evaluate its medical efficacy and long-term health effects.

- Fund research on cannabis-related disparities in Black men, including studies on racialized policing, economic barriers in the legal market, and health risks.

7. Workforce Development and Career Pathways

- Establish vocational training programs that prepare Black men for careers in the legal cannabis industry, including cultivation, dispensary operations, and regulatory compliance.

- Partner with Historically Black Colleges and Universities (HBCUs) and community colleges to create educational pathways into cannabis science, policy, and entrepreneurship.

8. Criminal Justice Reform and Public Safety

- Address racial disparities in post-legalization policing, ensuring that Black men are not disproportionately targeted for cannabis-related citations or impaired driving enforcement.

- Implement law enforcement diversion programs, redirecting individuals from incarceration to public health-based treatment options.

The Role of Community-based Organizations on Health

Community-based organizations (CBOs) play a pivotal role in addressing the healthcare disparities faced by Black men by implementing targeted interventions that enhance access to quality care and promote overall well-being.

Here are several ways CBOs can support this mission:

1. Health Education and Awareness Programs:

- **Chronic Disease Management**: Offer workshops and seminars on managing conditions prevalent among Black men, such as hypertension, diabetes, and cardiovascular diseases.

- **Preventive Care Promotion**: Encourage regular health screenings and check-ups to facilitate early detection and treatment of illnesses.

- **Artificial Intelligence**: Utilize mobile apps, social media, and AI-driven chatbots to disseminate preventive health education directly to Black men through accessible and relatable content. (Note: AI is not a substitute for justice; its deployment must be guided by ethical safeguards, accountability measures, and equity frameworks that protect vulnerable communities from bias and harm, in alignment with federal and international standards for responsible AI.)

2. Mental Health Support Services:

- **Culturally Humble Counseling**: Provide access to mental health professionals who understand and respect the cultural contexts of Black men.

- **Support Groups**: Establish safe spaces for Black men to discuss mental health challenges and share coping strategies. Collaborate with community-based businesses, such as barber shops, where Black men frequent to create support group types of initiatives.

- **Virtual Support**: Invest in culturally relevant digital mental health apps and virtual therapy services tailored for Black men, addressing stigma and improving access to care.

3. Advocacy and Policy Engagement:

- **Healthcare Policy Reform**: Advocate for policies that address systemic biases and improve healthcare access for Black men.

- **Funding for Research:** Push for increased funding dedicated to research on health issues disproportionately affecting Black men.

4. Workforce Development in Healthcare:

- **Medical Career Pathways:** Create programs that mentor and support Black men pursuing careers in healthcare to increase representation.

- **Training for Cultural Humility:** Offer workshops for existing healthcare providers to improve their understanding of the unique health needs of Black men.

5. Community Health Initiatives:

- **Mobile Health Clinics:** Deploy mobile units to provide healthcare services in underserved areas.

- **Partnerships with Local Organizations:** Collaborate with churches, fraternities, sororities, and other community groups to disseminate health information and services.

- **Centers for Medicare and Medicaid Services (CMS)**: Recognize the vital role of community health workers (CHWs) in enhancing patient care by introducing billable services for CHWs under Medicare Part B.

o   Develop Collaborative Training Programs: Hospitals can partner with educational institutions to create training curricula that equip CHWs with the necessary skills to address community-specific health challenges. For instance, the Laredo Public Health Department collaborated with Texas A&M International University's School of Engineering to enhance community health services through technology-driven solutions.

o   Integrate CHWs into Care Teams: Incorporating CHWs into multidisciplinary healthcare teams allows for comprehensive patient support. CHWs can bridge cultural and linguistic gaps, facilitate communication, and provide personalized care, leading to improved health outcomes.

o   Establish Community-based Learning Opportunities: Creating internships and field placements for CHWs within hospital settings provides hands-on experience and fosters a workforce adept at addressing diverse health needs.

o   Leverage New Medicare Billing Codes: Hospitals should utilize the new Medicare billing codes for community health integration services, ensuring that CHW services are financially sustainable. This includes conducting social drivers of health assessments and providing ongoing support services.

o   Engage in Policy Advocacy: Collaborating with CHW associations and other stakeholders to advocate for supportive policies can enhance the integration and effectiveness of CHWs in healthcare settings.

6. Addressing Social Drivers of Health:

- **Economic Empowerment Programs:** Enhance and implement individualized job training and placement services to improve economic stability, which is closely linked to health outcomes.

- **Safe Housing Initiatives:** Advocate for and develop affordable housing communities to ensure Black men have access to safe living environments.

By focusing on these areas, community-based organizations can make significant strides in removing barriers to quality healthcare and improving the physical and mental health outcomes for Black men. When we support Black men, we improve chronic disease outcomes for all high-risk groups, reduce emergency room visits, and relieve strain on overstretched health systems. Culturally humble mental health services for Black men also enhance care for veterans, immigrants, and rural residents who face similar stigmas and access barriers.

While physical and mental health disparities are pressing, they do not occur in a vacuum. The social and economic conditions in which Black men live—where they sleep, learn, work, and try to build futures—shape the very foundation of their health. To understand the root of these disparities, we must look beyond the clinic and into the structures that either support or suffocate opportunity. The following story captures the intersection of housing, education, and economic vulnerability—and how systemic inequities reverberate through every aspect of Black men's lives.

A John Henry Story: "Two Evictions and a Dream"

John Henry had always been good with his hands. Roofing, painting, hauling—you name it. After his father passed, he dropped out of community college to help support his mom and younger brother. He figured he would go back once things settled down. That was twelve years ago.

Now, at 36, he was on his second eviction notice in three years. Rent kept going up, even when the heat didn't work. His pay hadn't. His credit score was shot—not from overspending, but from emergencies: a busted transmission, a hospital bill from when his daughter had an asthma attack, a loan he co-signed on for a cousin who disappeared.

When he tried to apply for a mortgage, the banker looked at his zip code before his W-2s. "Maybe try again next year," they said, as if time was something he could afford.

Meanwhile, John Henry's son sat in a classroom with broken windows and outdated textbooks. His school didn't have AP classes, but it had a metal detector. John Henry wanted more for him—trade school, college, maybe tech. But how do you build dreams when you're busy trying to survive?

He wasn't asking for handouts. Just a chance. A loan that didn't come with predatory strings. A landlord who answered calls. A school that prepared, not punished. He wanted stability—not just for himself, but for the next John Henry coming up behind him.

Housing, Education, Broadband Access, and Economic Stability as Social Drivers of Health

"We carry the weight of dreams denied, but we also carry the keys to new doors." **- Jay Ellis**

Rooted in the SDOH framework, pillar two will take an intersectional approach that focuses on housing, education, broadband access, and economic stability.

Housing as a Social Driver of Health

- The United States is grappling with a severe housing crisis marked by rising unaffordability, increasing instability, and limited choices for marginalized groups[72]. This crisis has critical health implications, especially for marginalized communities. Studies[73] link housing conditions with various health outcomes, including chronic illness, mental health, maternal and infant health, and injury. Addressing housing issues

---

72 Housing as a determinant of health equity: A conceptual model
73 An Intersectional Approach to Social Determinants of Stress for African American Men: Men's and Women's Perspectives

comprehensively could serve as a vital pathway to reducing health inequities across social and economic groups.

- Homeownership is widely regarded as a cornerstone of the American dream and a key to building intergenerational wealth. This path is less accessible for Black Americans, who have a homeownership rate of 46.4%, compared to 75.8% for white families. Additionally, homes in predominantly Black neighborhoods are valued at $48,000 less than those in predominantly white areas, leading to a cumulative equity loss of approximately $156 billion[74].

In summary, the severe housing crisis in the United States, which disproportionately affects marginalized communities, not only limits economic opportunities for Black Americans but also exacerbates health inequities across social and economic groups, highlighting the urgent need for comprehensive housing reform to promote health and wealth equity.

Proposed Housing Policy Recommendations

The Brookings Institution proposed the following housing policy recommendations[75]:

- Increase support for small dollar mortgage loan programs.

- Reduce uneven costs of mortgages for Black homeowners.

- Extend credit and down payment assistance to borrowers impacted by discriminatory housing and lending practices.

- Adopt credit scoring practices with less discriminatory impacts.

---

74   Homeownership, racial segregation, and policy solutions to racial wealth equity
75   Homeownership, racial segregation, and policy solutions to racial wealth equity

- Increase diversity in the appraisal profession. Nearly nine in ten property appraisers are white, while 2% are Black, according to Urban Institute analysis of 2019 Census data.

- Consider using AI-driven tools to identify housing disparities and prioritize investments in affordable housing projects in historically marginalized communities.

- While artificial intelligence holds promise in addressing systemic inequities, its deployment must be accompanied by robust ethical guardrails—such as the AI Bill of Rights and NIST's Risk Management Framework—alongside regular audits for bias, strong data privacy protections, meaningful human oversight in high-stakes decisions, and clear transparency standards to ensure AI tools do not replicate or exacerbate the very disparities we seek to eliminate.

The Role of Community-based Organizations in Housing

- **100 Black Men of America**: This organization offers mentoring and support services that include housing assistance, aiming to improve the quality of life within African American communities.

- **National Urban League (NUL)**: NUL provides housing counseling and foreclosure prevention services to help Black men, and their families, secure and maintain affordable housing.

- **Church-based Initiatives**: Many Black churches run housing assistance programs, offering temporary shelter and support services to those in need.395

- **Non-profits and philanthropic entities**: Nonprofit and philanthropic organizations play pivotal roles in addressing societal needs and fostering community development.

A John Henry Story: "The Empty Desk"

John Henry was the kind of kid who loved questions. Why the sky changed colors. Why his mother had two jobs. Why his schoolbooks were taped at the seams while the kids across town had new Chromebooks and digital whiteboards.

In third grade, he raised his hand so much his teacher started calling him "Professor." But by seventh grade, the lights in his eyes had dimmed. The school counselor told him college might not be for "kids like him." When he asked for tutoring, there wasn't funding. When he asked about STEM programs, he was told to focus on behavior first.

By the time high school came around, John Henry had already seen more security guards than guidance counselors. When he skipped class, no one called home. When he showed up, the teachers looked surprised.

He graduated. Barely. And when he looked around the auditorium, he could count the number of Black boys on one hand. Most of the desks in his AP classes had been empty—because so few had ever made it that far.

Now, as a father, John Henry is determined to change the story for his son. But he still carries the weight of an education system that never saw his brilliance. All he wanted then—and now—is a fair shot.

Education as a Social Driver of Health

- It has long been established that education significantly influences health outcomes, serving as a key social driver of health[76]. Individuals with higher education levels often experience better health, including lower rates of chronic diseases and longer life expectancy. One study analyzing the impact of the *Affordable Care Act* revealed that, after 2014 (when the

---

76   Social Determinants of Health: Education Access and Quality

ACA was implemented), 44.0% of non-Hispanic White men aged 18 to 64 had attained some college education or higher, compared to 27.4% of their non-Hispanic Black counterparts[77]. The same study found that in the post-ACA era of 2015-2019, an estimated 15.3% of non-Hispanic Black men and 7.6% of non-Hispanic White men ages 18-64 were uninsured and an estimated 41.5% of non-Hispanic Black men and 30.2% of non-Hispanic White men ages 18-64 lacked a usual source of medical care.

- The relationship between education and health also operates through various pathways, where higher educational attainment often leads to better job opportunities, health insurance, and safer living environments, which collectively enhance health outcomes. However, according to the National Center for Education Statistics (NCES), in the 2021-22 academic year, Black men earned 3.0% of all doctoral degrees conferred to U.S. citizens and permanent residents, while white men earned 32.5%[78]. Similar disparities track along the K-12 and post-secondary education ecosystems[79].

- Research by Dr. Shervin Assari[80] and Dr. Darrell Hudson[81] shows that higher education and income do not offer the same health protections for Black men as they do for white men. Despite socioeconomic advancement, Black men face persistent discrimination and chronic stress, leading to higher rates of depression, hypertension, and other health issues. This "diminished returns" phenomenon reveals that education alone cannot overcome systemic racism's impact on Black men's health, reinforcing the need for structural change alongside educational and economic initiatives.

77   Examining the Impact of the Affordable Care Act on Access to Care for Black Men and White Men: Implications for Policy and Practice
78   National Center for Education Statistics
79   Racial Inequality in Education
80   Black men face high discrimination and depression, even as their education and incomes rise
81   The relationship between socioeconomic position and depression among a US nationally representative sample of African Americans

- Data from the National Center for Education Statistics (NCES) indicate that Black male students are less likely to enroll in and complete college compared to other racial groups. In 2019, about 27% of Black men aged 18 to 24 were enrolled in college, compared to 42% of white men in the same age group. NCES (2019) posit only half as many Black men have a Masters' degree (4%) as Black women (9%), white men (8%) and white women (13%). Of Black doctorate degrees earned, Black women account for 65%.

- In the 2020–2021 school year, Black, non-Hispanic men accounted for 1.3% of the nation's 3.8 million public school teachers, according to the National Center for Education Statistics National Teacher and Principal Survey. Overall, Black, non-Hispanic men are 6.1% of the general US population[82].

- Data from the National Center for Education Statistics indicates that Black students participate in at least one Career and Technical Education (CTE) course at a rate of 82%, comparable to their white peers. However, disparities emerge as students progress, with only 18% of Black students achieving CTE concentrator status (completion of three CTE courses), compared to 22% of white students[83].

- It has been well-established that the less education one possesses, the less likely they are to have high quality and/or employer-sponsored health insurance. One study analyzing the impact of the *Affordable Care Act* revealed that, after 2014 (when the ACA was implemented), 44.0% of non-Hispanic white men aged 18 to 64 had attained some college education or higher, compared to 27.4% of their non-Hispanic Black counterparts[84]. The same study found that in the post-ACA era of 2015-2019, an estimated 15.3% of non-Hispanic Black men and

---

82 How many Black male teachers are there in the US?
83 Advancing Racial Equity in Career and Technical Education Enrollment
84 Examining the Impact of the Affordable Care Act on Access to Care for Black Men and White Men: Implications for Policy and Practice

7.6% of non-Hispanic white men ages 18-64 were uninsured. Similarly, an estimated 41.5% of non-Hispanic Black men and 30.2% of non-Hispanic white men ages 18-64 lacked a usual source of medical care.

Proposed Education Policy Recommendations

Addressing the intertwined disparities in education and health outcomes, particularly among Black men, requires comprehensive policy interventions. The following recommendations aim to bridge these gaps:

- **Enhance Educational Access and Quality:**

  o **Early Childhood Education:** Invest in high-quality early learning programs to establish a strong educational foundation.

  o **K-12 Support:** Allocate resources to underfunded schools, implement mentorship initiatives, and provide academic support to improve graduation rates among Black male students.

  o **Higher Education Opportunities:** Offer scholarships, grants, and support services to increase enrollment and completion rates for Black men in post-secondary institutions.

  o **Virtual Access**: Expand access to virtual mentorship, e-learning, and digital upskilling platforms to help Black men build pathways to higher education and vocational success.

The Role of Community-based Organizations in Education

Community-based organizations (CBOs) play a pivotal role in enhancing educational outcomes for Black men, thereby positively influencing their health and economic stability. Their contributions include:

- **Black in AI**: An organization dedicated to increasing the presence of Black individuals in the field of artificial intelligence through workshops, mentorship, and networking opportunities.

- **100 Black Men of America**: Their Saturday Leadership Academy provides mentoring and educational support to young Black men, focusing on leadership development and academic achievement.

- **Fraternities and Sororities**: Various civic organizations offer scholarships, tutoring, and mentoring programs to support the educational advancement of Black men.

- **Non-profits and philanthropic entities**: Nonprofit and philanthropic organizations play pivotal roles in addressing societal needs and fostering community development.

A John Henry Story: "Disconnected"

John Henry had the skills. What he didn't have was WiFi.

He had found a promising job listing for a remote help desk role that paid better than anything in his neighborhood. But the application was online, the resume builder needed an update, and his cracked smartphone couldn't upload the file. The public library's computers were full. The hotspot from his cousin's old tablet timed out before he could hit submit.

His son's school had moved to hybrid learning, but the internet at home cut out every time someone streamed video. Homework turned into arguments. Virtual parent-teacher conferences were missed. And when John Henry tried to schedule a telehealth appointment for his anxiety, the platform wouldn't load.

He wasn't lazy. He wasn't unmotivated. He was disconnected—literally.

Every door he tried to walk through was locked behind a login screen. And every time he reached for opportunity, it felt like the signal dropped. All he needed was access—a decent connection, a working device, and someone to show him how to use it.

Because in this era, being offline meant being left behind.

Digital Access and Broadband Infrastructure

Why Broadband Access Matters

Access to reliable, affordable broadband Internet is no longer a luxury; it is a fundamental social driver of health. Broadband access directly impacts education, employment, healthcare, and civic engagement—critical areas that shape the well-being and opportunities of Black men. Yet Black communities are disproportionately affected by the digital divide. According to the Pew Research Center, as of 2021, nearly 29% of Black households lacked broadband access compared to 20% of white households.

For Black men, equitable access to broadband is crucial for:

- **Education**: Enabling participation in remote learning, technical training programs, and higher education

- **Economic Stability**: Accessing job applications, entrepreneurial resources, financial services, and online professional development

- **Healthcare Access**: Using telehealth and teletherapy services, particularly mental health resources tailored to Black men

- **Civic Engagement:** Registering to vote, staying informed on policy issues, and participating in digital organizing efforts

Without broadband access, existing disparities in health, education, and economic opportunity are exacerbated, deepening systemic inequities.

Proposed Digital Access and Broadband Infrastructure Policy Recommendations

- **Expand Federal and State Investment:** Increase funding for broadband infrastructure projects in historically underserved Black communities through programs such as the Broadband Equity, Access, and Deployment (BEAD) Program.

- **Subsidize Internet Access:** Provide vouchers, tax credits, or subsidies to low-income Black households to ensure affordable broadband services.

- **Support Community Digital Hubs:** Equip community-based organizations (e.g., churches, fraternities, sororities, nonprofits etc.) to serve as local hubs for free or low-cost Internet access, device lending, and digital literacy training.

- **Integrate Digital Skills Training:** Embed digital literacy, cybersecurity awareness, and online career readiness skills into educational and workforce development programs targeting Black men.

Alignment with Healthy People 2030

- ***Healthy People 2030* Objective:** Increase the proportion of individuals with broadband access.
- **Playbook Focus:** Ensure equitable digital access as a foundation for health, education, and economic mobility.

- Increase broadband subscription rates among Black households by 25% over four years.
- Expand telehealth utilization among Black men for physical and mental health services.
- Grow participation rates in digital literacy and technology training programs offered by community-based organizations.

The Role of Community-based Organizations in the Digital Access Ecosystem

Community-based organizations (CBOs) can play a pivotal role in closing the digital divide by:

- Hosting public WiFi hotspots and device loan programs
- Offering digital literacy classes tailored to Black men and boys
- Partnering with Internet service providers to secure discounted service plans for their communities
- Advocating at the local and state level for equitable broadband policies and investments

By strengthening broadband access and digital literacy, CBOs can help Black men unlock new pathways to educational attainment, economic stability, and improved health outcomes.

A John Henry Story: "The Side Hustle Never Sleeps"

John Henry woke up at 5:00 a.m.—again. He still had not slept more than four hours. His first job was a warehouse shift. The second was delivering groceries. The third was a dream deferred: a t-shirt printing business he was trying to build in the basement between exhaustion and responsibility.

His résumé was solid. Trade certifications. A clean record. Years of management experience. But the jobs that paid what he was worth either didn't call back or offered salaries far below market—when they saw his name, his address, his skin.

He had been laid off twice during the pandemic and burned through his savings trying to keep the lights on. His credit took a hit. He avoided the doctor even when his back seized up because he had lost health coverage. Every dollar he earned was a decision—gas or groceries, rent or rest.

He wasn't failing. The system was. And despite the degrees and the grind, the stress had started creeping into his body: migraines, blood pressure spikes, nights spent pacing instead of dreaming.

John Henry didn't need a handout. He needed a path. One that didn't punish him for being Black and working hard. One that recognized that economic stability isn't just about money—it's about health, dignity, and the freedom to breathe.

Economic Stability as a Social Driver of Health

- Black men have long been excluded from economic and wealth-building opportunities. Because of structural racism, Black men have historically been more likely to be unemployed compared to white men[85]. During the COVID-19 pandemic, the typical duration of unemployment among Black men was 20.1 weeks, compared with 16.6 weeks among white men. In 2020, Black men earned just 75 cents for every $1 earned by white, non-Hispanic men[86].

- It has also been well-documented that socioeconomic status is a "fundamental cause" of disease. By shaping access to

---

85   Systemic and Structural Racism: Definitions, Examples, Health Damages, and Approaches to Dismantling
86   Black Men and the U.S. Economy: How the Economic Recovery Is Perpetuating Systemic Racism

essential resources, these factors influence a variety of health outcomes through multiple pathways and continue to be linked with disease[87].

- A recent study found that in 2018, the economic impact of racial and ethnic health disparities was estimated at $421 billion, and health inequities linked to educational differences were estimated to cost $940 billion dollars[88].

- Despite higher incomes and higher education, Black men are more likely to experience depression and anxiety[89].

A John Henry Story: "Breathless on Both Ends"

The air felt heavy that day, thicker than usual. The fans in John Henry's apartment pushed warm air in circles while his son, Jamal, lay on the couch wheezing. The asthma pump was nearly empty, and the pharmacy said the insurance lapsed. Again.

Their window faced the expressway, where trucks passed day and night. When the breeze blew in, it carried more dust than relief. A smokestack from the old plant down the block puffed out something gray every morning. Some days, John Henry swore it settled in his chest.

The neighborhood had no trees, no shaded parks. Just cracked sidewalks, asphalt, and heat. Summers were brutal. His electric bill doubled each July, and when he couldn't pay, the A/C went off. Jamal once passed out walking home from school. The ER doctor blamed dehydration, but John Henry blamed the zip code.

---

87   Social conditions as fundamental causes of disease
88   The Economic Burden of Racial, Ethnic, and Educational Health Inequities in the US
89   For Black men, higher education and incomes don't lower risks of depression, researchers say

He remembered his grandmother's stories of front porches and fresh air. His family had moved here for opportunity. Instead, they got proximity— to pollution, to heat, to silence.

John Henry didn't choose to live next to diesel fumes and concrete. But choices were limited. Rent was "affordable." The price, though, was paid in migraines, inhalers, and rising temperatures.

He wanted to breathe. That's it. Just breathe easy—for himself, for his son, for his block.

Environmental Justice and Climate Resilience

Environmental factors are deeply intertwined with economic stability and health equity. Black men are disproportionately exposed to environmental hazards—living near industrial plants, highways, landfills, and other pollution-intensive sites—which increases the risk of chronic illnesses such as asthma, cancer, and cardiovascular disease according to the Centers for Disease Control and Prevention and the Environmental Protection Agency.

In urban areas, many predominantly Black neighborhoods also function as urban heat islands, where a lack of tree canopy and green spaces significantly elevate temperatures during the summer. This contributes to higher rates of heat-related illnesses and hospitalizations, particularly among older adults, children, and individuals with pre-existing health conditions, according to the Centers for Disease Control and Prevention.

Research[90] shows that air pollution in California's San Joaquin Valley alone costs the economy roughly $3 billion annually—about $1,000 per resident—through premature deaths, asthma attacks, school absences, and lost workdays. Freight emissions, which disproportionately

---

90   California Partnership for the San Joaquin Valley Air Quality Workgroup

impact Black and Hispanic neighborhoods, generate nearly $47 billion each year in transportation-related public health damages[91]. Historically redlined communities—often majority-Black—suffer shorter life expectancies (by 3.6 years on average, and up to 21 years in some cities) and face greater risks from climate-driven hazards, including insurance coverage loss due to "bluelining[92]."

In places like Louisiana's "Cancer Alley," Black residents are exposed to chloroprene at levels more than 700 times the national average, creating both lethal health risks and lasting financial hardship[93]. These compounding costs—healthcare bills, lost wages, reduced property values, and diminished wealth-building opportunities—make environmental justice a core economic stability issue, demanding urgent, targeted policy solutions.

To address these disparities, targeted interventions are essential:

- Collaborate with policymakers, public health departments, and urban planners to monitor and reduce environmental exposure in Black communities.

- Launch urban greening and tree-planting campaigns to reduce heat exposure, improve air quality, and enhance neighborhood health and livability.

- Expand energy assistance and weatherization programs to mitigate the financial burden of extreme temperatures, which drive up electricity and gas bills due to increased reliance on heating and air conditioning systems.

These environmental inequities are not only health threats—they also impose financial burdens that further entrench systemic disadvantage. Proactively addressing climate resilience and environmental

---

91   Environmental injustice in America: Racial disparities in exposure to air pollution health damages from freight trucking
92   Is Bluelining the 'New' Redlining? How Insurance Discrimination Deepens Climate Disparities
93   Toxic tensions in the heart of 'Cancer Alley'

justice is critical to building healthier, more sustainable, and economically stable communities for Black men and their families.

Proposed Economic Stability Policy Recommendations

To address the economic disparities and health inequities affecting Black men, the following policy recommendations are proposed. More in-depth economic stability recommendations can be found in the appendix:

1. Enhance Employment Opportunities

- **Targeted Job Training Programs**: Develop and fund vocational training and apprenticeship programs specifically designed for Black men, focusing on high-demand industries (Informational Technology, Quantum Computing, Cybersecurity, etc.) to improve employability and reduce unemployment rates.

- **Subsidized Employment Initiatives**: Implement subsidized job programs that provide temporary wage support to employers hiring Black men, facilitating entry into the workforce and gaining valuable experience.

- **Artificial Intelligence**: Deploy AI-based job matching platforms that connect Black men to stable employment opportunities and entrepreneurship support based on skills and interests.

2. Promote Wage Equity

- **Strengthen Anti-discrimination Enforcement**: Enhance the capacity of agencies like the U.S. Equal Employment Opportunity Commission (EEOC) to enforce anti-discrimination laws effectively, ensuring fair wages and addressing systemic biases in compensation.

- **Support Unionization Efforts:** Encourage and protect the rights of Black men to unionize, as union membership has been shown to reduce wage disparities and improve working conditions.

3. Facilitate Wealth-building

- **Access to Capital for Entrepreneurship:** Expand access to capital through grants, low-interest loans, and forgivable loan programs for Black entrepreneurs to foster business ownership and wealth accumulation.

- **Financial Literacy Programs:** Implement community-based financial education initiatives to equip Black men with the knowledge to manage finances, invest, and build wealth effectively.

4. Improve Health Outcomes

- **Integrate Health and Economic Policies:** Recognize the link between economic stability and health by designing policies that simultaneously address employment, income, and health disparities.

- **Mental Health Support Services:** Increase funding for mental health services tailored to Black men, addressing higher rates of depression and anxiety despite socioeconomic advancements. Collaborate with organizations with missions to support Black mental health such as Black Psychiatrists of America.

5. Enhance Data Collection and Research

- **Disaggregated Data Analysis:** Mandate the collection and analysis of data on employment, wages, and health outcomes disaggregated by race, gender, socioeconomic status and other intersectional characteristics to identify specific disparities and inform targeted interventions.

- **Community-based Participatory Research**: Support research initiatives that involve Black men in the study design and implementation processes to ensure culturally relevant and effective policy solutions.

Implementing these policies requires collaboration between federal, state, and local governments, private sector stakeholders, and community organizations to create a comprehensive approach that addresses the multifaceted challenges faced by Black men in achieving economic stability and health equity.

The Role of Community-based Organizations on Economic Stability

Community-based Organizations (CBOs) play a pivotal role in enhancing the economic stability of Black men by addressing systemic barriers and promoting equitable opportunities. Here are several strategies these organizations can implement:

- **Job Training and Employment Programs**: Develop tailored vocational training and apprenticeship programs that align with current market demands, ensuring Black men acquire skills for stable, well-paying jobs. For instance, the 100 Black Men of Greater Washington, D.C., in collaboration with Wells Fargo, offers the Pathways to Success program, focusing on workforce readiness and creating pipelines for corporate careers and entrepreneurial endeavors.

- **Financial Literacy and Wealth-building Initiatives**: Provide workshops on budgeting, saving, investing, and credit management to empower Black men with the knowledge to build and sustain wealth. Implement digital financial literacy programs and mobile budgeting tools to empower Black men with real-time financial management strategies. The Black Economic Alliance is an example of a coalition committed to driving economic equality for Black people by leveraging collective expertise and networks.

- **Entrepreneurship Support**: Offer resources such as business development workshops, mentorship, and access to capital to encourage and support Black men in starting and growing their own businesses. Organizations like the National Urban League provide such support through various programs aimed at economic empowerment.

- **Advocacy for Equitable Employment Practices**: Engage in policy advocacy to address discriminatory hiring practices and promote fair wages. The NAACP, for instance, works to eliminate race-based discrimination and ensure the health and well-being of all persons.

- **Mental Health Support Services**: Recognize the link between economic stress and mental health by providing access to counseling and support groups tailored to the experiences of Black men. Churches and fraternities often offer such support within the community.

- **Networking and Mentorship Opportunities**: Create platforms for Black men to connect with professionals and mentors who can provide guidance, support, and opportunities for career advancement. Fraternities and sororities have established mentorship programs that serve this purpose.

- **Housing Assistance Programs**: Assist in securing affordable housing, which is foundational to economic stability. Community development corporations (CDCs) often focus on providing housing solutions in underserved communities.

Health and Wellness Programs

Implement initiatives that address health disparities, recognizing that good health is essential for economic productivity. By implementing these strategies, community-based organizations can significantly contribute to the economic stability and overall well-being of Black men, addressing both immediate needs and systemic inequities. Additionally, we stimulate economic growth, increase tax contributions, and decrease dependency on public assistance. Job training and housing access strategies designed for Black men also help other underserved populations, including working-class white men, Latino men, and returning citizens.

In addition to these broad strategies, there are exemplary organizations already embodying this mission in action. Two such models—the Black Executive Men Community and the Monumental Men's Network—demonstrate how targeted, high-impact networks can translate economic empowerment principles into measurable outcomes. As a founding member of the Monumental Men's Network, I have seen firsthand how intentional leadership development, mentorship, and strategic relationship-building can accelerate economic mobility for Black men. These organizations not only create pathways to professional success but also strengthen the economic and civic foundations that underpin health equity.

Civic Engagement, Violence Prevention, and Fatherhood Support as Social Drivers of Health

"Politics impacts you whether you want it to or not." **Joy-Ann Reid**

Pillar three emphasizes community empowerment and civic engagement, violence prevention, and fatherhood programs. Contextually, recognizing the growing national focus on the challenges faced by men and boys, several state governors have initiated programs to address these issues. In Maryland, Governor Wes Moore has directed (as of this writing in 2025) state agencies to develop targeted solutions for uplifting men and boys. Michigan's Governor Gretchen Whitmer has signed an executive directive to boost young men's participation in higher education and skills training. Connecticut's Governor Ned Lamont is working to increase male representation in K-12 teaching positions, and Utah's Governor Spencer Cox has established a Task Force on the Wellbeing of Men and Boys.

These initiatives underscore a bipartisan commitment to addressing the systemic challenges affecting men and boys, aligning with the objectives of the *John Henry Health Equity Playbook* to promote health equity and community empowerment. On July 30, 2025, Governor Newsom issued an executive order directing California's Health and Human Services Agency to develop a coordinated statewide response

aimed at reducing suicides among young men and boys by strengthening mental health supports, combating stigma, and creating pathways
to education, work, mentorship, and community connection.

Moreover, the Commission on the Social Status of Black Men and Boys
(CSSBMB)[94] was established through bipartisan legislation passed by
Congress and signed into law in August 2020. Sponsored by former
Senator Marco Rubio (R-FL) and Rep. Frederica Wilson (D-FL), this
landmark initiative underscored a rare moment of cross-party unity
to address the urgent and systemic disparities facing Black men and
boys in the United States. This should not be about partisan politics, it
should be about ensuring equitable representation at the local, state,
and federal levels.

The Commission operates under the U.S. Commission on Civil Rights
and is tasked with examining the social conditions impacting Black
males—including disparities in education, health, economic opportunity, criminal justice, and fatherhood. It issues policy recommendations
to Congress, the White House, and federal agencies aimed at eliminating these disparities.

This bipartisan framework aligns with the core values of the *John Henry
Health Equity Playbook* by demonstrating that advancing the well-being of Black men is not a partisan issue but a national imperative. The
CSSBMB serves as a successful precedent and a structural model for the
playbook's proposed initiatives, such as the establishment of a Federal
Office of Men's Health and the expansion of community-based interventions to support economic mobility, fatherhood, and health equity.

Just as the CSSBMB brought together diverse leaders across the political spectrum to advocate for meaningful, evidence-based policy
change, this playbook calls for sustained, bipartisan investment in the
health and future of Black men. As former Senator Rubio stated, "the
disparities that disproportionately affect Black men and boys in America are not a partisan issue—they're an American issue."

---

94   United States Commission on the Social Status of Black Men and Boys

A John Henry Story: "The Line That Never Moved"

John Henry arrived at the polling place before sunrise, coffee in one hand and his voter registration card in the other. He had checked his status twice online just to be sure. This was his first time voting in a midterm election, and he wanted his voice to count.

But the line snaked out the door and down the block, past the shuttered grocery store and the corner where the bus never came on time. An hour passed. Then two. The woman ahead of him left to pick up her kids. A man behind him left for work. Poll workers moved slowly, apologizing but explaining there was only one functioning voting machine for the entire precinct.

When John Henry finally reached the table, they told him his name wasn't on the list. "Must be a mistake," he said, pulling up the confirmation email on his phone. The poll worker handed him a provisional ballot. No explanation. No guarantee it would be counted.

Walking out into the afternoon sun, John Henry thought about the roads that got paved in other neighborhoods, the schools that got better funding, and the clinics that stayed open. He thought about who made those decisions—and how easy it was to keep people like him out of the process.

That day, he realized voting wasn't just about showing up. It was about the fight to stay in line, to be seen, to be counted. And it was a fight he wasn't willing to lose.

Empowering Black Men Through Civic Engagement

Civic engagement, including the right to vote, is not only a democratic cornerstone but also a critical determinant of health and well-being.

Ensuring that Black men are empowered to actively participate in the political process will enhance their visibility in policymaking, allow them to advocate for equitable resources, and foster healthier, more resilient communities. Voting and political participation enable Black men to influence policies that affect their health, economic opportunities, and social conditions, addressing the systemic barriers that have historically marginalized them.

Why Voting Matters for Health Equity

Research underscores a strong link between civic engagement and community health outcomes. According to the Healthy Democracy Healthy People initiative, communities with higher voter participation rates experience better health outcomes, as voting influences decisions on healthcare, environmental protections, social services, and education funding. When Black men participate in elections at all levels—local, state, and federal—they can help shape policies that address health disparities, increase access to quality healthcare, and promote economic stability.

A Note on Gerrymandering and Its Impact on Civic Participation

While access to the ballot is essential, the power of that vote also depends on fair representation. Gerrymandering undermines this principle by manipulating district boundaries in ways that can silence Black communities and diminish their influence on the policies that shape health, economic opportunity, and public safety.

Gerrymandering[95]—the manipulation of electoral district boundaries to favor one political party—has profound implications for Black communities, particularly Black men. By diluting voting power through "packing" (concentrating voters of color into a few districts) or "cracking" (splitting them across multiple districts), gerrymandering reduces political representation, undermines the ability to elect candidates

---

95   What to Know About Redistricting and Gerrymandering

who reflect community priorities, and weakens advocacy for policies that address health equity, economic stability, and public safety.

For Black men, whose health and well-being are directly shaped by policy decisions, diminished representation can mean fewer investments in community-based health services, housing, education, and violence prevention. As gerrymandering becomes a permanent feature of political strategy, protecting fair maps is not only about today's elections but about safeguarding the voice, representation, and long-term health and economic futures of Black men and the generations that follow.

Therefore, addressing gerrymandering requires a multi-pronged approach: establishing independent redistricting commissions, adopting clear and transparent mapping criteria, increasing public participation in map-drawing, and enforcing the *Voting Rights Act* to ensure that district lines do not dilute the electoral influence of communities of color.

Strategies to Enhance Political Participation

Sustained political power—and the health equity it can help secure—requires moving beyond one-off election drives to a continuous, community-rooted process. This model blends proven voter engagement tactics with a five-phase cross-cycle strategy, ensuring that Black men and their supporters are informed, organized, and mobilized in ways that address both systemic barriers and local priorities. It integrates education, barrier reduction, strategic partnerships, community organizing, and data-driven outreach into a seamless year-round plan.

For instance, organizations such as Win With Black Men, Black Male Voter Project, Million Man Vote, the Health Alliance Network, Black Men Vote, and others provide strong models for operationalizing elements of this cross-cycle civic engagement plan -- demonstrating how sustained organizing, culturally grounded outreach, and strategic partnerships can strengthen political power and advance health equity for Black men. The goal is to engage in short-term tactics while playing the long game in terms of strategy.

The Cross-Cycle Civic Engagement Plan

This model is designed to operate continuously across **all levels of elections**—local (school boards, city councils, mayoral races), state (legislatures, governors), and federal (Congressional midterms and presidential elections). While presidential races often generate the most visibility, the same cycle repeats at every level, ensuring Black men's voices and priorities are carried into each arena of decision-making. This approach facilitates meaningful and sustained relationship-building that ensures engagement is not reduced to one-off transactions, particularly when working with historically marginalized populations.

Phase 1: Listen & Assess (Post-presidential Election to Quarter 2 of Non-election Years)

- Build trust through listening sessions, barbershop conversations, and community surveys.
- Identify top local issues, mapping concerns by values cluster and neighborhood.
- Begin forging partnerships with advocacy organizations such as the NAACP Legal Defense Fund, Million Man Vote, and local community groups to lay the groundwork for year-round engagement.
- **Outcome:** Clear community priorities and strategic alliances that will guide sustained civic action.

Phase 2: Educate & Build Base (Quarter 3–Quarter 4 of Non-election Years)

- Launch targeted education campaigns—including podcasts, social media series, and in-person forums—on the importance of voting and its direct connection to health equity.

- Leverage community leaders, faith-based organizations, and advocacy partners to disseminate information widely.
- Teach residents to interpret sample ballots, understand school board authority, and follow city council decision-making.
- **Outcome:** Informed community members who understand both the mechanics and stakes of civic participation.

Phase 3: Organize & Inspire (6–9 Months Before an Election)

- Run storytelling campaigns such as "Why I Vote" to connect personal narratives to policy impact.
- Distribute sample ballots and issue scorecards that highlight how small races affect daily life, public health, and economic stability.
- Use mobile apps and digital platforms to educate about ballot measures, streamline registration, and encourage participation in local, state, and federal elections.
- **Outcome:** Motivated voters who see the direct stakes of participation and feel equipped to act.

Phase 4: Mobilize to Vote (Last 90 Days Before Election)

- Host voter registration pop-ups, barbershop/salon voter days, and voter health fairs.
- Provide transportation to polls, resources for early voting, and assistance navigating voting requirements to reduce barriers such as restrictive ID laws or limited polling locations.
- Emphasize the importance of voting in all races—up and down the ballot—and how these decisions shape community health outcomes.
- **Outcome:** Higher turnout among Black men and allied voters in targeted districts.

Phase 5: Hold Leaders Accountable (Immediately After Election)

- Share voter turnout data, community wins, and areas for improvement.
- Host "We Voted—Now What?" events to set expectations for elected officials and sustain momentum.
- Publicize scorecards tracking whether campaign promises align with actions, leveraging advocacy partners to maintain public pressure.
- **Outcome:** A culture of accountability that strengthens long-term community power and policy impact.

Institutionalizing Voting and Civic Engagement as Health Equity Tools

Sustaining these efforts requires institutionalizing civic engagement within the framework of health equity. By advocating for the inclusion of voting rights in health policy discussions, this agenda aims to establish civic participation as an essential element of health equity strategies for Black men. A civically engaged Black male community will not only have greater political power but also create a healthier, more equitable society where policies reflect the needs and voices of Black men.

Organizations like the Black Executive Men Community and Monumental Men's Network build more than professional networks—they nurture civic leaders. Members gain tools to influence policy, serve on boards, and mobilize communities, transforming individual career success into collective civic power. By integrating leadership development with policy advocacy, these networks help ensure that Black men's voices and experiences shape decisions that affect health, wealth, and opportunity.

- **Voter Participation as a Public Health Objective**: In June 2023, the Office of Disease Prevention and Health Promotion

(ODPHP) designated voter participation as a 'core objective' in the nation's health goals, *Healthy People 2030*. This recognition underscores the link between civic engagement and health outcomes.

- **Impact of Voting on Health Policies:** Voting influences decisions on critical health-related issues, including Medicaid expansion, public health funding, and policies addressing social determinants of health. Increased voter turnout in marginalized communities can lead to policies that more effectively address their health disparities.

- **Barriers to Voting:** Structural barriers such as voter ID laws, limited polling locations, and disenfranchisement disproportionately affect marginalized populations, including Black men. These barriers can diminish their political influence and hinder progress toward health equity.

By integrating strategies to promote voting and civic engagement into health equity initiatives, public health professionals can help ensure that policies reflect the needs and voices of marginalized communities, thereby advancing health equity.

A John Henry Story: "The Corner that Changed Everything"

John Henry never liked that corner. It was the one you had to pass on the way to the bus stop, the one with the boarded-up liquor store and the group of young men posted up—passing time, passing bottles, passing looks. He would nod, keep moving, and hope the day stayed quiet.

One summer evening, the quiet broke. Two cars screeched to a stop. Shouts. A flash. Then the sound—sharp, deafening, final. Everyone scattered. John Henry ducked behind a dumpster, his heart pounding so hard it felt like it might crack his ribs.

The sirens came late.

The tape went up fast.

And the next morning, the corner looked the same—except for the candles and a photo of a boy who had just made varsity basketball. John Henry didn't know him well, but he knew his story: too few jobs, too many guns, not enough safe spaces.

That night, John Henry sat on his porch, thinking about his own son. He wanted him to know more than survival. He wanted him to know opportunity, mentorship, and the feeling of being safe walking down his own street.

He realized violence prevention wasn't just a police matter, it was a community matter. It was about giving young men better options than that corner. Options that could change everything.

Violence Prevention

Black men are at a higher risk of homicide, face barriers to mental health services, and experience trauma that can have lifelong impacts. Addressing these challenges requires a comprehensive, trauma-informed approach that empowers Black men and strengthens community bonds.

- **Elevated Homicide Rates:** Homicide is a leading cause of death among Black men aged 15 to 34, accounting for nearly 40% of gun homicides in the U.S., despite this group comprising just 2% of the population[96].

- **Barriers to Mental Health Services:** Black men are less likely to seek or receive appropriate mental health care due to factors such as implicit bias among healthcare providers, economic

---

96   Community-based Violence Interruption Programs Can Reduce Gun Violence

constraints, lack of insurance, and limited availability of culturally competent providers[97].

- **Lifelong Impact of Trauma**: Exposure to violence, systemic racism, and socioeconomic hardships contributes to complex trauma among Black men, leading to increased risks of depression, anxiety, post-traumatic stress disorder, chronic stress-related physical health issues, and intergenerational effects impacting family dynamics[98].

- **Violence Prevention Efforts**: Community-based violence intervention (CVI) programs have shown promise in reducing gun violence among Black men. For instance, the implementation of violence interruption programs was associated with a 63% decrease in gun shooting victimization in South Bronx, New York, and a 43% reduction in gun-related deaths and assaults in Richmond, California[99].

Addressing these challenges requires comprehensive strategies, including community-based interventions, policy reforms, and efforts to enhance cultural competence among healthcare providers.

Proposed Violence Prevention Policy and Practice Recommendations

1. Community-driven Approaches

- **Engage Black Men as Leaders in Prevention**: Encourage Black men to take active roles in violence prevention efforts as mentors, community organizers, and peer advocates. This can involve establishing community councils where Black men can lead discussions on violence, strategize solutions, and create support systems.

---

97   Intimate Partner Violence Prevention Resource for Action
98   Programs and Services for Black Male Survivors of Community Violence: What's Effective?
99   Community-based Violence Interruption Programs Can Reduce Gun Violence

- **Promote Trauma-informed Care and Healing Spaces**: Communities can benefit from trauma-informed care models that acknowledge the specific stressors Black men face due to historical and ongoing discrimination. Programs should provide safe spaces for Black men to access mental health support and trauma recovery resources. Collaborate with mental health providers who are trained in Eye Movement Desensitization and Reprocessing (EMDR) and other types of trauma treatments to support brothers in these healing spaces.

2. Address Social Drivers of Violence

- **Economic Stability and Job Opportunities**: Addressing poverty and unemployment through job training programs, small business support, and mentorship initiatives for Black men can reduce economic drivers of violence.

- **Educational and Skill-building Programs**: Equip Black men with conflict resolution, financial literacy, and life skills to help them navigate challenging situations without resorting to violence.

3. Policy and Legislative Advocacy

- **Support Gun Violence Prevention Policies**: Work with policymakers to advocate for policies aimed at reducing gun violence, including background checks, safe storage laws, and firearm training programs. The policy should prioritize community safety while respecting constitutional rights.

- **Invest in Youth Development Programs**: Advocate for funding of youth development and mentorship programs that provide positive outlets for young Black men, reducing pathways to violence.

4. Strengthening Community Resources and Partnerships

- **Community Policing and Trust Building**: Encourage police departments to work closely with Black communities to build trust, engage in bias training, and foster respect. Transparency in policing can help prevent violence and create an environment where Black men feel safer and more supported.

- **Public Health and Medical Support**: Partner with healthcare providers to implement screenings for violence risk factors and connect Black men to mental health resources, social services, and substance use treatment when necessary.

5. Data Collection and Research

- **Collect and Share Data on Violence Prevention Efforts**: Reliable data on violence among Black men can guide targeted interventions and improve program effectiveness. Regularly collect, analyze, and share data with stakeholders to identify successful strategies and areas for improvement.

- **Predictive Analytics**: Apply predictive analytics to identify violence hotspots and deploy targeted community-based interventions, while also ensuring that such technologies are used equitably and with community consent.

- **Support Participatory Research**: Include Black men in research on violence prevention to ensure that their voices, needs, and experiences shape interventions and outcomes.

Implementation and Monitoring

- **Evaluation Metrics**: Develop metrics to track the success of violence prevention efforts in Black communities, including reductions in violence-related injuries and deaths, improvements in mental health, and community perceptions of safety.

- **Community Feedback**: Establish mechanisms to gather feedback from Black men and community members regularly. Incorporate their insights into program adjustments and policy recommendations.

Preventing violence against Black men is critical for advancing health equity, fostering safer communities, and breaking cycles of trauma and adversity. By implementing community-driven, culturally responsive strategies, providing economic and social support, and advocating for protective policies, we can empower Black men and create environments where they thrive. The *John Henry Health Equity Playbook* advocates for collective action and ongoing collaboration with Black men as equal partners in violence prevention, reinforcing their role as change agents and leaders in community safety.

A John Henry Story: "The Sound in the Night"

John Henry woke to the sound—sharp, echoing through the summer air. One. Two. Three pops. Then silence. He lay still, listening for the return of quiet, for the signal that it was over. Somewhere outside, tires screeched, a car door slammed, and the night swallowed the noise.

He had heard it before. Too many times. On the walk to the bus stop. From his porch on a Friday night. Outside the corner store where he grabbed coffee each morning. But each time, it was different. Each time, he thought about the mothers, the friends, the faces that wouldn't be at church on Sunday.

Last year, his cousin Marcus didn't make it home. Wrong place, wrong time. The funeral program listed his age—22. John Henry thought about how Marcus never got the chance to vote, to start the welding business he had been saving for, to see his little sister graduate.

John Henry knew this wasn't just about "bad neighborhoods" or "bad decisions." It was about jobs that never came, schools that closed, empty lots that stayed empty, and laws that looked the other way. It was about the air you breathed, the street you lived on, and whether the world thought your life was worth protecting.

Gun violence doesn't just steal lives, it steals futures.

Gun Violence as a Public Health Issue

Gun violence is a critical public health issue in the United States, disproportionately affecting Black men. Understanding this disparity through the lens of social drivers of health—such as economic stability, education, social and community context, health care access, and neighborhood environment—is essential for developing effective interventions[100].

Black men are disproportionately affected by gun violence, experiencing significantly higher firearm-related homicide rates compared to white men. For Black men aged 15 to 24, firearm homicides exceed all other leading causes of death, including accidents, suicide, heart disease, and cancer[101]. The statistics below are provided by the Everytown for Gun Safety Support Fund and the Violence Policy Center unless otherwise cited:

- Homicide was the leading cause of death in 2018 with 95.2% involving guns for Black men aged 15-24.

- From 2018 to 2021, the average gun homicide rate for Black men was 45.7 deaths per 100,000 people, compared to 2.7 for white

---

100   Gun Violence and Public Health: A Crisis We Can't Ignore
101   Childhood trauma and neighborhood disorder impact mental health of injured Black men

men. This means Black men were over 17 times more likely to die by gun homicide than white men during this period[102].

- In 2018, the gun homicide victimization rate for Black males (34.22 per 100,000) was more than 14 times higher than for white males (2.40 per 100,000).

- Every 11 minutes, a Black American is shot and wounded, and every three hours, a young Black man dies by gun homicide in the United States.

- In Illinois, Black people are 34 times as likely as white people to die by gun homicide[103].

- Black Americans account for 81 percent of the victims in the 50 cities with the highest murder rates, despite making up only 38 percent of the population in those cities.

Proposed Gun Violence Policy and Practice Recommendations

To address gun violence among Black men effectively, a multifaceted approach targeting the underlying social drivers is necessary:

1. **Invest in Economic Development**: Enhancing economic opportunities in predominantly Black communities can reduce violence. This includes job creation, workforce development programs, and support for Black-owned businesses.

2. **Improve Educational Opportunities**: Access to quality education can serve as a protective factor against involvement in violence. Policies should focus on equitable funding for schools, mentorship programs, and pathways to higher education.

---

102   The Changing Demographics of Gun Homicide Victims and How Community Violence Intervention Programs Can Help
103   Illinois Gun Sales and Violence Persist Heading into Fourth of July Weekend

3. **Enhance Community-based Violence Intervention (CVI) Programs**: Implementing programs that mediate conflicts and provide support services can effectively reduce gun violence. For instance, Baltimore's Group Violence Reduction Strategy offers resources to individuals at risk, contributing to a significant decrease in homicides. The Everytown Community Safety Fund supports and invests in CVI programs, recognizing their importance in reducing gun violence.

4. **Expand Access to Mental Health Services**: Providing culturally competent mental health care can help address the trauma associated with exposure to violence. This includes community-based counseling and support groups.

5. **Implement Sensible Gun Policies**: Enforcing background checks, restricting access to firearms for individuals with a history of violence, and regulating firearm sales can reduce gun-related incidents.

6. **Foster Community Engagement and Trust**: Building trust between law enforcement and Black communities through community policing and accountability measures can improve cooperation and safety.

7. **Address Environmental Factors**: Improving neighborhood conditions by addressing blight, increasing green spaces, and ensuring safe recreational areas can reduce crime rates and improve residents' quality of life.

By addressing the social drivers of health, these policy and practice recommendations aim to reduce gun violence and improve the overall well-being of Black men in the United States.

A John Henry Story: "The Saturday Morning Ritual"

Every Saturday morning, before the city awoke, John Henry and his eight-year-old son, Caleb, would hit the park with a basketball and a backpack full of snacks. Caleb dribbled awkwardly, his small hands working overtime to keep the ball from bouncing away. "Bend your knees," John Henry would say, demonstrating the shot. The ball sailed, bounced off the rim, and Caleb laughed—a laugh so full it seemed to hang in the crisp morning air.

This was their ritual. No phones. No rush. Just father and son, moving through a game that was less about points and more about presence. They talked about dinosaurs, math homework, and why the clouds looked different in the fall. Sometimes, Caleb asked about the scar on John Henry's hand from his welding days. Sometimes, he asked harder questions—about why some kids didn't have a dad at home, or why his father had to work nights.

John Henry didn't shy away. He told Caleb the truth—about hard work, about mistakes, about showing up even when it wasn't easy. He knew his presence was more than just a comfort. It was a foundation. A living, breathing rebuttal to every headline, statistic, and stereotype that tried to paint fathers like him as missing.

For John Henry, fatherhood wasn't an obligation, it was an anchor.

Fatherhood: Supporting Black Men as Fathers

"Being present is revolutionary. In a world that expects us to disappear, showing up is an act of love and resistance."
- Dr. Michael Eric Dyson

Fatherhood is a pivotal role that shapes families, communities, and society. For Black men, the journey of fatherhood is often met with unique challenges due to systemic inequities and societal stereotypes. Supporting Black fathers in their roles benefit children, strengthens families, and empowers communities. Black fatherhood in the United States is a multifaceted subject that challenges many prevailing stereotypes.

Contrary to common misconceptions, a significant proportion of Black fathers are actively involved in their children's lives, regardless of their living arrangements. Father involvement is associated with multiple family health benefits, including improved child development, emotional well-being and mental health. This section provides actionable strategies and policy recommendations to support Black men in becoming actively involved, informed, and empowered fathers.

Living Arrangements and Involvement:

- Approximately 59.5% of Black fathers reside with their children, equating to about 2.5 million out of 4.2 million Black fathers[104].
- Among those who live with their children, Black fathers are notably engaged in daily activities[105]:
- 70% bathe, diaper, or dress their children daily, compared to 60% of white fathers and 45% of Hispanic fathers.
- 35% read to their children daily, surpassing 30% of white fathers and 22% of Hispanic fathers.

Non-resident Fathers:

- Even when not residing with their children, Black fathers maintain substantial involvement:
- 67% see their children at least once a month, higher than 59% of white fathers and 32% of Hispanic fathers[106].

Challenges and Societal Factors:

- Black fathers often face systemic challenges, including higher incarceration rates and economic disparities, which can impact family dynamics. Despite these obstacles, many remain committed to their parental responsibilities[107].

These insights underscore the importance of recognizing and supporting the diverse experiences of Black fathers, moving beyond stereotypes to appreciate their significant contributions to their families and communities.

---

104   Debunking the most pervasive myth about Black fatherhood
105   6 Actual Facts Shatter the Biggest Stereotypes of Black Fathers
106   6 Actual Facts Shatter the Biggest Stereotypes of Black Fathers
107   The Absent Black Father: Race, the Welfare-Child Support System, and the Cyclical Nature of Fatherlessness

Proposed Fatherhood Support Policy Recommendations

1. **Promoting Positive Father-child Relationships**

    o **Encourage Quality Time**: Advocate for policies that support parental leave, enabling fathers to spend essential bonding time with their children, especially during critical early developmental stages.

    o **Community Programs for Engagement**: Support the creation and funding of fatherhood programs within communities that foster father-child bonding through structured activities and workshops. These programs, like those championed by the National Fatherhood Initiative, can help fathers learn about child development, emotional bonding, and age-appropriate parenting strategies.

2. **Enhancing Economic Stability and Employment Opportunities**

    o **Job Training and Employment Support**: Offer workforce development programs tailored to fathers, especially those recently out of incarceration or facing employment barriers. Emphasize job readiness, skill-building, and access to stable jobs.

    o **Access to Financial Literacy Resources**: Financial stress can be a barrier to fatherhood engagement. Support programs that provide Black fathers with resources on budgeting, managing credit, and planning for future expenses. ACF's Responsible Fatherhood program emphasizes financial literacy as a crucial component of responsible parenting.

3. **Strengthening Healthy Co-parenting and Family Dynamics**

    o **Healthy Relationship Education**: Promote education on conflict resolution and communication for fathers, encouraging them to maintain healthy relationships with co-parents, which can reduce stress and provide a stable environment for children.

o **Family Counseling Services**: Support initiatives that fund family counseling, helping fathers navigate relationships, parenting stresses, and co-parenting dynamics effectively.

o **Virtual Support**: Develop online fatherhood support communities and mobile parenting resources specifically designed for Black fathers, offering culturally resonant content on parenting, mental health, and co-parenting skills.

4. **Breaking Down Systemic Barriers to Fatherhood Engagement**

o **Advocate for Legal Reforms**: Fathers often face legal barriers related to custody, child support, and visitation. Champion legal reforms that enable fathers to maintain consistent, positive involvement in their children's lives.

o **Community-based Support Networks**: Encourage partnerships with community organizations that provide mentorship and support for Black fathers, offering guidance on parenting, navigating legal issues, and balancing responsibilities.

5. **Promoting Mental and Physical Well-being**

o **Mental Health Resources for Fathers**: Advocate for accessible mental health resources, including culturally competent therapists, specifically targeting stressors Black fathers face. Support policies that provide affordable mental health services.

o **Health Screenings and Wellness Programs**: Fatherhood creates a strong motivation for men to prioritize their health, helping them move beyond harmful stereotypes that discourage preventive care and encouraging greater engagement in their well-being for the sake of their families. Include fathers in health and wellness initiatives by capitalizing on their frequent intersection with healthcare as caregivers in pediatric and obstetric clinical spaces.

Conclusion

Fatherhood is an opportunity to promote the health of men because they have a new and strong motivation to remain healthy for their families. Supporting Black fathers strengthens families, reduces inter-generational disparities, and fosters a healthier, more resilient society. By empowering Black men as fathers, we contribute to a future where every child can thrive, secure in the guidance, love, and support of their fathers. When we support Black men, we strengthen families, increase voter turnout, and build safer, more engaged communities. Father-hood initiatives for Black men can potentially reduce ACEs (Adverse Childhood Experiences) and contribute to better long-term health and academic outcomes for children of all backgrounds[108]. The next section will discuss the unique role of male engagement and paternal support.

---

108   Adverse Childhood Experiences in a low-income Black cohort: The importance of context

A John Henry Story: "In the Delivery Room"

John Henry still remembers the feeling of the hospital chair beneath him—hard plastic, barely comfortable—but he wouldn't have traded that seat for anything in the world. His wife, Maya, was in active labor, gripping his hand so tightly that his knuckles turned white. The room was a blur of monitors, beeping machines, and medical staff speaking in terms that seemed just out of reach. John Henry leaned in close, steadying her breathing with his own, whispering reminders that she was strong, that she was safe, and that he wasn't going anywhere.

When the nurse suggested a procedure Maya wasn't sure about, John Henry didn't hesitate. He asked questions. He translated the jargon. He reminded the team of her birth plan. It wasn't confrontation, it was advocacy. And in that moment, Maya's shoulders relaxed just a little.

The tension eased.

The room slowed down.

Later, as he held his newborn daughter, skin to skin, John Henry understood something he hadn't before. This role—father, partner, advocate—wasn't just about love. It was about power. The kind of power that comes from being informed, present, and prepared to fight for the well-being of the people you love most.

He wondered how many other fathers wanted to be this prepared but didn't know where to start. How many needed training, resources, and encouragement to step into that delivery room not just as bystanders, but as active partners in care. For John Henry, the answer was clear; if men could be trained to build bridges or lead work crews, they could be trained to support life at its most critical moment.

Paternal Support and Doula Training as Health Equity Strategies

Too often, maternal health conversations exclude the vital role of fathers. Expanding maternal health to include *male engagement and paternal support* is an emerging public health imperative. Research shows that when Black men are informed, engaged, and supported throughout the prenatal and postpartum periods, the entire family benefits—especially mothers and infants.

Despite systemic barriers, Black fathers continue to show strong involvement. In fact, a CDC study found that Black fathers living with their children were more likely than white or Hispanic fathers to engage daily in caregiving and family activities—such as bathing, changing, or dressing their children, sharing meals, and helping with homework[109]. Yet their formal inclusion in perinatal health programs, including doula training, remains rare. Community-based paternal doula models—where men are trained to support birthing individuals—can advance health equity by reducing maternal stress, improving birth outcomes, and fostering stable family units. At the end of this section, you will find a few "Dad doula-related" programs as a reference.

Why It Matters

- **Maternal Stress and Birth Outcomes:** Fathers who are engaged during pregnancy contribute to lower rates of low birthweight and premature births.

- **Intergenerational Health:** Early paternal involvement influences infant development, reduces toxic stress, and sets the stage for long-term health and educational success.

- **Culturally Aligned Support:** Black male doulas, or father-focused doula programs, can build trust and address the

---

109   Fathers' Involvement With Their Children: United States, 2006–2010

historical mistrust Black communities have toward the healthcare system.

- **Mental Health Impacts:** Both parents are vulnerable to *postpartum depression* and related mental health challenges, especially in under-resourced environments. Untreated postpartum depression in either parent can disrupt bonding, emotional regulation, and family stability.

Key Data

- The National Responsible Fatherhood Clearinghouse reports that engaged fathers are associated with fewer maternal depressive symptoms and better child outcomes.

- A 2022 *Maternal and Child Health Journal* study found that paternal involvement during prenatal care correlated with a 13% reduction in the likelihood of low birthweight.

- According to the CDC, up to 1 in 10 men experience postpartum depression, yet most remain undiagnosed or untreated due to stigma and lack of awareness.

- HealthConnect One and the National Black Doulas Association have promoted community-led support models that include culturally responsive mental health education.

Proposed Paternal Support Policy Recommendations

1. **Fund Paternal Doula Training Programs**

   o Allocate grants to community-based organizations to create culturally competent doula training programs that include or are led by Black men.

2. **Integrate Fathers into Maternal Health Initiatives**

   o   Mandate father-inclusive perinatal health strategies as part of Medicaid Managed Care contracts and maternal mortality prevention plans.

3. **Expand Research and Data Collection**

   o   Fund studies on the impact of male doulas and paternal support on maternal and infant outcomes to build the evidence base.

4. **Promote Early Fatherhood Education**

   o   Invest in school- and community-based programs that prepare young men for healthy relationships and future parenting roles.

5. **Promote Mental Health Awareness and Normalize Support**

   o   Launch campaigns that promote awareness of postpartum depression in both mothers and fathers, destigmatize mental health care, and normalize help-seeking behaviors—especially among Black men. These campaigns should highlight that postpartum mental health is a shared family concern, not just a maternal issue.

6. **Ensure Access to Affordable, Culturally Humble Mental Health Care**

   Expand access to affordable, culturally humble mental health providers through Medicaid expansion, loan forgiveness for providers serving in shortage areas, and mobile/telehealth mental health services. Black men and fathers must have low-barrier access to professionals who understand their lived experiences and unique stressors.

Alignment with *Healthy People 2030* Objectives

- Reduce the rate of maternal mortality (MICH-04).
- Increase the proportion of pregnant women who receive early and adequate prenatal care (MICH-10).
- Increase the proportion of parents who use positive parenting practices (EMC-02).
- Increase the proportion of people with depression who receive treatment (MHMD-04).

A Few Featured Dad Doula Programs & Initiatives

Dads to Doulas (St. Louis & Virtual)

A six week curriculum created by Dear Fathers, founded by Brad Edwards and Kyra Betts. It equips Black men and expectant fathers with advocacy skills, education on pregnancy, birth physiology, perinatal mood disorders, and infant care to improve maternal and infant outcomes. The program launched in 2024 and continues growing today.

Dad Doula University (Milwaukee & Virtual)

Founded by Joshua Liston-Zawadi in 2021, this program offers free workshops for non-birthing parents to navigate emotional changes, pregnancy, and personal growth. It is delivered virtually and now at the Sherman Phoenix Marketplace. Graduates receive certification, keepsakes, and essentials like diapers.

Fathers Assisting Mothers (FAM) – Dad Doula Bootcamp (Kansas City)

Led by James Hogue, this nonprofit offers the "Dad Doula Bootcamp" and "DadPrep Academy" to prepare expectant fathers to support their birthing partners proactively—responding to elevated maternal risks and the lack of male doula representation.

Hey Black Dad (New Jersey)

Founded by Peter Bullock, this in-person and virtual doula service supports men through prenatal, birth, and postpartum stages—providing tools tailored to Black fathers' experiences.

Conclusion

To achieve true maternal and family health equity, Black fathers must be viewed as essential participants—not afterthoughts. Doula training, mental health support, and perinatal engagement for Black men are transformative, evidence-based strategies that can foster stronger families, reduce disparities, and promote holistic healing. Health systems must intentionally include and uplift Black men as co-creators of family wellness—not merely as support staff, but as full partners in care and community change.

Four-year Plan

Year 1: Establishing a Health Equity Infrastructure for Black Men Through Executive Order

1a. Support the Launch of the National Health Equity Initiative for Black Men

Why: Using executive order as a start, this initiative aims to tackle chronic diseases disproportionately affecting Black men as established in the literature. The National Institute on Minority Health and Health Disparities (NIHMD) has highlighted the importance of tailored prevention and intervention strategies for historically marginalized populations like Black men, further justifying this as a top priority. Culturally-sensitive promotion of healthy eating, physical activity, and medical help-seeking behavior would be commensurate with this effort. Further, enacted legislation like the *Commission on the Social Status of Black Men and Boys Act* (with consequent convenings of the Commission Taskforce) provides additional context for supporting the unique needs of Black men.

Addressing health inequities for Black men requires a holistic approach that incorporates housing, education, and economic stability. Each of these domains significantly influences health outcomes, and targeting these areas can yield both direct and indirect improvements in health.

Metrics: Reduction in various diseases (e.g., heart disease, cancer, diabetes, sickle cell anemia, etc.) among Black men; increased access to preventive services and mental health care.

Incorporating NIMHD Research Priorities: NIMHD's focus on eliminating health disparities through precision medicine and community-based interventions will inform the implementation of this initiative, ensuring that it is data-driven and tailored to the unique health profiles of Black men.

1b. Expand Access to Mental Health and Substance Use Disorder Services

Why: Mental health services are critically underutilized by Black men due to stigma, lack of culturally humble care, and access barriers. Quantitative and qualitative studies underscore the role of systemic barriers in preventing Black men from accessing care, and the NIMHD has similarly identified mental health as a key area of disparity. The initiative will also address barriers to mental health services, a critical issue given that only 26.4% of Black adults with mental illness receive treatment. Expanding access through community-based mental health programs and mobile health units will help overcome these barriers.

Metrics: Increase in the number of Black men receiving mental health services; reduction in mental health stigma; improved mental health outcomes such, as reduced depression and suicide rates. Increase in the number of Black men receiving treatment; reduction in overdose deaths; improved recovery rates.

Incorporating NIMHD Research Priorities: NIMHD research underscores the importance of culturally relevant interventions. Mental health programs will include culturally competent training for providers and public health messaging that resonates with Black men, reducing stigma and encouraging care utilization.

2a. Build Wealth by Expanding Homeownership and Affordable Housing Opportunities for Black Men

Why: The severe housing crisis in the U.S. has immediate and significant health impacts, particularly among marginalized communities and is linked to chronic conditions, mental health, and other issues. Addressing housing can thus serve as a crucial first step to reducing health disparities and building a stable foundation for addressing education and economic stability. Given the unique housing barriers Black men face, prioritize interventions that increase access to affordable rental housing, support homeownership, and combat discriminatory practices in lending and appraisals.

Metrics: Housing affordability index, homeownership rates by race, rental affordability, mortgage approval rates.

2b. Supporting Educational and Vocational Pursuits for Black Men as a Pathways to Economic and Social Mobility

Why: Supporting the educational aspirations of Black men is essential for addressing long-standing disparities in health, housing, and economic stability. Education serves as a critical social driver of health, with higher educational attainment strongly correlated by better health, greater economic security, and access to stable housing. Despite making up 6.1% of the U.S. population, Black men are significantly underrepresented in higher education and critical professions, including only 3.0% of all doctoral degree earners and 1.3% of the nation's public school teachers.

Vocational education and training (VET) offer a practical pathway to bridge these gaps. VET programs equip individuals with specific skills tailored to industry demands, facilitating quicker entry into the workforce and providing opportunities for stable, well-paying jobs. For Black men, engaging in vocational pursuits can lead to immediate employment, reducing unemployment rates and fostering economic stability. Data from the National Center for Education Statistics indicates that

Black students participate in at least one Career and Technical Education (CTE) course at a rate of 82%, comparable to their white peers. However, disparities emerge as students progress with only 18% of Black students achieving CTE concentrator status (completion of three CTE courses), compared to 22% of white students.

Without targeted support, Black men face barriers to education, limiting their access to quality job opportunities, health insurance, and safe living conditions—all of which contribute to poorer health outcomes and economic vulnerabilities. Addressing these educational disparities is crucial not only for enhancing individual potential but for promoting intergenerational stability and resilience in Black communities.

Metrics: Enrollment rates across the education ecosystem for Black men, mentorship program participation and outcomes, vocational outcomes, graduation rates, access to education resources, job placement rates, employer retention rates, uninsured rates for Black men, chronic disease prevalence (e.g., hypertension, diabetes, etc.) among Black men across education levels, Black male representation in high-demand, high-income industries (e.g., tech, finance, real estate).

3. Propose and Pass a *Black Entrepreneur Loan Forgiveness Act* to Expand Access to Black Men's Business Grants and Technical Assistance Programs

Why: Financial stability is a social driver of health. Economic empowerment through forgivable loans to Black entrepreneurs will address wealth disparities and improve long-term health outcomes. Supporting Black men through business grants and technical assistance (i.e., Small Business Administration, Minority Business Development Agency) will enhance entrepreneurial success and contribute to closing the racial wealth gap. These resources will help Black men gain access to capital, mentorship, and the necessary skills to build sustainable businesses.

Metrics: Increase in Black men-owned businesses; access to and utilization of technical assistance programs; growth in business revenue and job creation within Black-owned businesses. Number of loans distributed; growth in Black-owned businesses; increase in household incomes among Black men.

First 100 Days: All Politics in Local

What are the differences between lobbying and advocacy[110]?

The John Henry Health Equity Playbook **is intended to inform, educate, and inspire. It does not constitute legal advice.**

Lobbying: The IRS describes lobbying as efforts to sway legislation by encouraging contacts with lawmakers or advocating for or against legislative measures. However, educational activities like holding meetings, distributing materials, or discussing public policy in an informative way are not classified as lobbying by the IRS.

Advocacy: The Lerner Center for Public Health defines public health advocacy as strategic actions aimed at influencing social, organizational, or policy changes to support health goals. This advocacy involves various activities, including coalition building, sharing evidence-based solutions, and lobbying, though lobbying is only one aspect of public health advocacy.

To be clear, according to IRS rules for 501(c)(3) organizations, general education about policy issues—such as what this playbook offers—is not lobbying. Lobbying refers specifically to attempts to influence legislation (e.g., urging a yes/no vote on a specific bill).

- **Lobbying at the Federal Level**: Advocate for the immediate establishment of the Office of Men's Health by engaging Congressional allies, such as members of the Congressional

---

110   Politics and Public Health Playbook: Strategies for Public Health Institutes and Their Partners

Black Caucus. Emphasize the policy's alignment with NIMHD's research findings on health disparities.

- **State-level Action**: Partner with state legislators in regions with high Black male populations (e.g., the South, as identified in recent studies) to push for Medicaid expansion and enhanced funding for community-based health initiatives.

- **Local Engagement**: Mobilize city councils to adopt local health equity initiatives aligned with the national agenda, focusing on funding mobile health units and mental health outreach in underserved communities.

Midterm Election Strategy

- **Engagement Timeline**:

  o **12-18 months prior**: Mobilize constituents to raise awareness of key health and economic issues.
  o **6-12 months prior**: Host town halls and forums with local leaders to build momentum for midterm elections.
  o **3-6 months prior**: Activate grassroots lobbying efforts and run social media campaigns to push health equity priorities to the forefront of election debates.

- **Localized Voter Outreach**: Focus on issues specific to each state or district, prioritizing both urban and rural voters. Engage in grassroots efforts such as local events, canvassing, and digital outreach.

- **Emphasize Election Integrity**: Highlight transparent voting processes to counteract skepticism. Consider bipartisan endorsements to strengthen public confidence.

- **Digital Mobilization**: Leverage social media and data-driven insights to reach younger voters, encouraging early voting and registration.

- **Legal Readiness**: Prepare for election disputes with legal teams positioned to address recounts or other procedural concerns.

- **Adapt Messaging to Current Trends**: Tailor campaign themes around emerging issues, such as economic stability, climate change, healthcare, and public safety, with messages that resonate at a local level.

- **Data Utilization**: Use recent polling and demographic data to identify swing districts and optimize GOTV efforts, adjusting strategies based on early voting and engagement metrics.

Year 2: Building Upon a Health Equity Infrastructure for Black Men

1. Establish a Federal Office of Men's Health

Why: Addressing the health disparities and inequities that Black men face, including higher rates of cardiovascular disease, prostate cancer, mental health challenges, and other chronic diseases, is a critical national priority. This dedicated office (that could be established by executive order) within the Department of Health and Human Services (HHS) will oversee research and policy development to improve Black men's health outcomes. This policy aligns with years of quantitative[111] and qualitative findings[112] regarding persistent gaps in access to care for Black men compared to White men. Establishing this office, as proposed by the *Men's Health Awareness and Improvement Act* addresses both structural discrimination and the invisibility of Black men in health research, as highlighted in quantitative and qualitative studies and reinforced by NIMHD research priorities.

Establishing a Federal Office of Men's Health will require bicameral legislative support and bipartisan leadership. This playbook calls for collaboration across both chambers of Congress and both parties

---

111   Examining the Affordable Care Act on Access to Care for Black Men and White Men: Implications for Policy and Practice

112   Giving Voice to Black Men: Guidance for Increasing the Likelihood of Having a Usual Source of Care

to institutionalize health equity for Black men as a federal priority. Importantly, as of May 1, 2025, the newly launched (for the 119th Congress) bipartisan Congressional Men's Health Caucus—co-chaired by Congressman Troy Carter (D-LA) and Congressman Rich McCormick (R-GA)—provides a critical policy window and legislative partner to advance men's health equity through initiatives like the proposed Federal Office of Men's Health.

Another strategy is to establish an interagency taskforce like the Property Appraisal and Valuation Equity (PAVE) Taskforce [113]. The federal office of men's health taskforce should include local, state, and federal stakeholders and employ a shared governance approach to ensure that all voices are heard. Convene hearings to provide for quantitative and qualitative data collection and policy recommendations to help shape what a federal Office of Men's Health can look like.

Metrics for success: Establishment of the office in year two supported by enacted legislation like the *Men's Health Awareness and Improvement Act* and a strategic plan to address men's health disparities; partnerships with research institutions for targeted research, particularly in states that have not expanded Medicaid, which studies have identified as exacerbating coverage gaps for Black men.

Incorporating NIMHD Research Priorities: The federal Office of Men's Health will coordinate with NIMHD to leverage insights from minority health research, ensuring that culturally appropriate interventions are prioritized. The office will also focus on addressing the intersectionality of race and gender, a critical point from studies and NIMHD's ongoing research.

As noted earlier, efforts to prioritize Black men's health must not come at the expense of women's health, family well-being, or gender equity. This is not a zero-sum game. We believe in solidarity. We believe in the power of community. And we believe that achieving true health equity

---

113   Action Plan to Advance Property Appraisal and Valuation Equity Closing the Racial Wealth Gap by Addressing Mis-valuations for Families and Communities of Color

means uplifting all people by addressing the unique needs of different populations, including men.

Just as the historic investment in women's health has brought forth transformative outcomes, so too can a focused effort to improve men's health infrastructure elevate the health of families and communities as a whole. Gender equity requires us to understand that neglecting one group harms us all. Men's health equity is family health equity. When fathers, brothers, and sons are healthy—physically, mentally, and emotionally—families are stronger, communities are safer, and public health systems are more resilient.

Our call to establish Offices of Men's Health is not an attempt to divert resources. Instead, it is a step toward inclusive equity, one that complements ongoing efforts to improve women's health. We envision a future where all people, regardless of gender, can thrive. That future begins with naming the gaps, investing in the solutions, and standing in solidarity across identities.

2. Institutionalize Voting and Civic Engagement as Health Equity Tools

Why: Civic engagement, including voting, is essential for securing and maintaining health equity initiatives. Ensuring that Black men participate fully in the political process will sustain long-term policy changes.

Metrics: Increase in voter registration and turnout rates; sustained advocacy efforts leading to health-related policy changes.

3. Implement Gun Violence Prevention Programs

Why: Gun violence is a major public health issue for Black men, particularly in urban areas. Community-based violence intervention and stricter gun control policies are needed to curb the epidemic.

Metrics: Reduction in gun-related deaths and injuries; increased participation in violence intervention programs.

Year 3: Empowering Fathers, Strengthening Families: Advancing Health and Stability for Black Men

1. Support Fatherhood and Family Stability Programs

Why: Engaging fathers early and often in their children's lives and supporting stable family structures improve both mental and physical health outcomes for Black men and their families.

Metrics: Increase in fatherhood program participation; improved family health outcomes; reduction in adverse childhood experiences (ACEs).

2. Ensure the Sustainability of the Office of Men's Health

Why: The Office of Men's Health will continue to oversee research, policy development, and programming to ensure that Black men's health remains a national priority.

Metrics: Increased funding for research on Black men's health; continued collaboration with public health agencies and research institutions.

Year 4: Sustaining Health Equity Progress

Overview:

Year four represents a critical turning point: the transition from building and scaling initiatives to embedding them sustainably across systems. In this final phase of the initial *John Henry Health Equity Playbook* roadmap, the priority shifts to institutionalizing gains, evaluating impact, ensuring accountability, and preparing for the next generation of Black men's health equity efforts.

Strategic Objectives:

1. **Institutionalize and Expand the Federal Office of Men's Health**

   o **Why:** Establishing the Office was a major milestone, but sustained leadership and dedicated funding streams are necessary to ensure longevity, bipartisan support, and integration across federal agencies (e.g., HHS, CDC, NIH, CMS).

- o **How:**

  - □ Advocate for permanent, mandatory appropriations (versus discretionary funding).
  - □ Embed men's health equity goals into agency strategic plans and grant funding priorities.
  - □ Establish regional Office of Men's Health hubs in partnership with HBCUs, community health organizations, and local governments.

- o **Metrics:** Federal funding secured; number of regional hubs established; integration of Black men's health into agency objectives and federal health research priorities.

2. **Evaluate and Strengthen Programs Launched in Years 1–3**

- o **Why:** Measurement ensures that progress is real, equitable, and scalable. It also helps demonstrate Return on Investment (ROI) to policymakers, funders, and communities.

- o **How:**

  - □ Commission independent evaluations of major initiatives (e.g., fatherhood programs, violence prevention programs, mental health access expansion).
  - □ Collect and publish disaggregated data (race, gender, age) to assess outcomes.
  - □ Hold community accountability sessions to report progress and refine strategies based on feedback.

- o **Metrics:** Evaluation reports completed; percentage of programs achieving stated goals; community satisfaction scores.

3. **Advance Local and State-level Policy Replication**

   o   **Why:** Sustained health equity progress requires scaling beyond the federal level. State and local governments are powerful actors in health policy implementation.

   o   **How:**

   □   Develop a *Black Men's Health Policy Toolkit* based on playbook strategies.
   □   Support the establishment of state and municipal Offices of Men's Health, modeled after the federal office and potential District of Columbia pilot.
   □   Advocate for the adoption of targeted universalism frameworks within state public health plans.

   o   **Metrics:** Number of states and cities adopting Black men's health initiatives; state-level legislation modeled on playbook strategies; partnerships formed with local CBOs and public health departments.

4. **Sustain Civic Engagement as a Health Equity Tool**

   o   **Why:** Civic engagement is health. Ensuring Black men's sustained participation in democracy protects long-term investments in health equity.

   o   **How:**

   □   Build permanent civic health coalitions linking voting, policy advocacy, and health initiatives.
   □   Continue targeted voter registration, education, and turnout campaigns aligned with major election cycles (presidential, midterm, local).
   □   Advocate for election policies that remove barriers and expand access (e.g., automatic voter registration, restoration of voting rights).

o   **Metrics:** Black men's voter registration and turnout rates; number of civic coalitions formed; number of health policies influenced through advocacy.

5. **Launch the John Henry Health Equity Fellowship Program**

o   **Why:** To sustain progress, leadership pipelines must be developed that nurture future advocates, policymakers, researchers, and health practitioners committed to advancing Black men's health equity at the local, state, and federal levels. As of this writing, a John Henry Institute for Black Men's Health and Policy Innovation has been established to catalyze these types of efforts (www.enyiastrategies.com)

o   **How:**

  □   Partner with HBCUs, medical schools, schools of public health, and professional organizations.
  □   Provide paid fellowship opportunities focusing on policy development, research, and community engagement.
  □   Prioritize fellows who demonstrate a commitment to culturally humble, asset-based approaches to Black men's health.

o   **Metrics:** Number of fellows recruited and graduated; fellow placement in leadership roles; fellow contributions to advancing policy and research agendas.

Conclusion

The John Henry Health Equity Playbook offers a transformative, actionable roadmap to confront the deeply entrenched health disparities impacting Black men, leveraging the enduring symbolism of John Henry's resilience to drive systemic change. Through a strategic, multi-dimensional approach that addresses healthcare access, economic stability, and civic empowerment, the playbook makes clear that targeted policies and community-driven solutions are essential to achieving sustainable progress.

As we move forward, this agenda issues a direct call to funders, policymakers, and business leaders: the cost of inaction is staggering. Racial and ethnic health disparities cost an estimated $421 billion from the U.S. economy annually with education-related health inequities adding another $940 billion in losses.

Black men's health disparities—preventable and deeply rooted in systemic barriers—represent both a moral failure and a missed economic opportunity. Investing in Black men's health and economic stability is not just the right thing to do, it is a strategic investment in America's future competitiveness, workforce productivity, healthcare cost containment, and community vitality. Men's health equity is community health equity. It is not a redistribution of care, but a reinvestment in people, too long overlooked. *The John Henry Health Equity Playbook* bridges the moral and business cases for urgent action, offering a clear, measurable, and high-return pathway to dismantle structural inequities and build a stronger, healthier, and more prosperous nation for all.

Appendix

The Political Determinants of Health Framework

The political determinants of health refer to the ways in which politics, policies, and political systems influence health outcomes and shape health inequities. This framework explores how laws, regulations, and government decisions impact social determinants of health, such as access to healthcare, education, housing, economic stability, and environmental conditions, which, in turn, affect individual and community health.

Key components of the political determinants of health include:

1. **Policy Decisions**: Government policies can either promote or hinder health equity. In this case, decisions about healthcare funding, Medicaid expansion, and public health initiatives directly affect access to care and the resources available for disease prevention and treatment.

2. **Legislation**: Laws that address issues such as environmental protection, labor rights, housing, and criminal justice reform have a significant impact on the social conditions that determine health outcomes. Policies that perpetuate systemic inequities can exacerbate health disparities.

3. **Political Power and Representation**: The distribution of political power influences whose voices are heard in policy debates and whose needs are prioritized. Communities with less political representation or influence are often left out of decision-making processes that affect their health and well-being.

4. **Voting and Civic Engagement**: Access to voting and political participation is a key determinant of health, as it allows communities to advocate for policies that promote health equity. Voter suppression and disenfranchisement can prevent marginalized populations from influencing health-related policies.

5. **Advocacy and Lobbying**: Health outcomes are also shaped by the advocacy efforts of various interest groups, including healthcare organizations, pharmaceutical companies, and public health advocates. These groups often lobby for or against policies that can either improve or harm public health.

The political determinants of health emphasize that health disparities are not just a result of individual behaviors or biological factors but are deeply rooted in the political environment. By addressing the political determinants, we can work towards achieving health equity and reducing health disparities across different populations.

The Commonwealth Fund Racial Equity and Policy-making Framework

The framework from the Commonwealth Fund, "Engaging the Voice to Support Racially Equitable Policymaking," focuses on involving historically marginalized communities in policymaking to advance racial equity.

Key elements include:

1. **Centering Community Voices**: Policies must be informed by those most affected by systemic inequities, ensuring their lived experiences are central to the policy process.

2. **Equitable Policy Design**: Policymakers should use data disaggregated by race and ethnicity to identify disparities and design interventions that target structural inequities.

3. **Power Sharing**: True equity requires shifting power dynamics so that communities of color have a meaningful role in decision-making, including leadership roles.

4. **Sustainable Engagement**: Policymaking should include long-term engagement and relationship-building with communities to foster trust and ensure policies evolve with their needs.

5. **Accountability Mechanisms**: Implement systems that hold policymakers and institutions accountable for equitable outcomes, including continuous monitoring and assessment of the policies' impacts on racial disparities.

The Centers of Disease Control and Prevention Social Determinants of Health Framework

Key social determinants are organized into five domains:

1. **Economic Stability**: Focuses on improving economic conditions to reduce poverty and increase financial security, which directly affects health.

2. **Education Access and Quality**: Enhances educational opportunities, recognizing that higher education levels correlate with healthier lifestyles and improved access to healthcare.

3. **Healthcare Access and Quality**: Seeks to improve healthcare availability and quality, ensuring all populations receive the necessary care to prevent and manage diseases.

4. **Neighborhood and Built Environment**: Prioritizes creating safe, accessible, and resource-rich environments that promote active lifestyles and minimize exposure to health hazards.

5. **Social and Community Context**: Emphasizes building supportive social networks and reducing discrimination and social isolation, which contribute to stress and poor health.

The framework underlines the need for policies and community initiatives that address these domains collaboratively. The CDC highlights that achieving health equity requires tackling SDOH to eliminate health disparities, reduce preventable conditions, and improve life expectancy across all demographic groups.

The Targeted Universalism Framework

1. **Establishing a Universal Goal**: Start by defining a clear, overarching objective that applies to everyone, such as equitable health outcomes or educational attainment.

2. **Assessing Barriers Across Groups**: Recognize that different groups face distinct obstacles based on social, economic, and structural conditions. This step involves a detailed analysis of the different ways people are positioned within social systems.

3. **Tailoring Strategies to Groups' Needs**: Develop targeted interventions that address the specific needs of each group, helping them overcome their specific challenges. This approach contrasts with "one-size-fits-all" policies, which often fail to address systemic disparities.

4. **Implementing with a Universal Approach**: The strategies work toward achieving the universal goal for all, but they are adaptable and context-specific, allowing flexibility to meet people where they are.

5. **Monitoring and Adjusting**: Regular assessment and adjustment ensure that interventions remain effective across diverse groups, adapting to changing social conditions or shifting needs.

Benefits of Targeted Universalism:

- **Equity-Focused**: It focuses on achieving equity by addressing unique systemic barriers, creating pathways for all groups to meet universal goals.
- **Inclusive**: Rather than singling out one group, the approach considers the needs of all, promoting broad-based support for equity-focused policies.
- **Adaptive**: It is dynamic and responsive to real-time data and evolving social dynamics.

In essence, Targeted Universalism is about recognizing that while all groups deserve equal outcomes, achieving those outcomes requires distinct, tailored interventions that address the specific contexts of each group. This approach provides a balanced framework for advancing policy goals that are both inclusive and equity-driven.

The Role of Artificial Intelligence (AI) and Machine Learning (ML)

Artificial Intelligence (AI) refers to the capability of computer systems to perform tasks that typically require human intelligence, such as reasoning, learning, perception, and problem-solving. These systems are designed to mimic cognitive functions associated with the human mind. Machine Learning (ML) is a subset of AI that focuses on developing algorithms enabling computers to learn from and make decisions or predictions based on data. Instead of being explicitly programmed for specific tasks, ML systems improve their performance as they are exposed to more data over time.

The federal government has provided guidelines for the responsible use of artificial intelligence[114]. Artificial intelligence holds significant potential to address health inequities, particularly among Black men, by enhancing economic opportunities, improving living environments, and mitigating biases in healthcare and education.

Here's how AI can be integrated into these areas:

1. Address Social Drivers of Health:

- **Economic Opportunities:**

    o **Job Training and Employment Programs**: AI-driven platforms can offer personalized job training by analyzing individual skills and matching them with market demands, thereby increasing access to stable, well-paying jobs with health benefits.

    o **Entrepreneurship Support**: AI tools can assist Black entrepreneurs in business planning, market analysis, and financial management, fostering economic stability within communities.

- **Safe Living Environments:**

    o **Community Development Projects**: AI can analyze crime patterns and environmental data to inform community development initiatives, leading to safer neighborhoods and better access to recreational facilities.

    o **Housing Improvements**: AI models can predict housing deterioration and prioritize areas for renovation, ensuring healthier living conditions.

---

114   Blueprint for an AI Bill of Rights

2. Implement Bias and Cultural Humility Training:

- **Healthcare Providers:**

    o **Bias Detection in AI Tools:** Develop AI algorithms that identify and mitigate biases in clinical decision-making processes, ensuring equitable treatment for all patients.

    o **Cultural Humility Training:** AI-powered simulations can provide healthcare professionals with scenarios to improve cultural sensitivity and address implicit biases.

- **Educational Institutions:**

    o **Inclusive Curriculum Development:** AI can analyze educational content to ensure it reflects diverse perspectives, promoting an inclusive learning environment.

    o **Personalized Learning:** AI-driven platforms can tailor educational experiences to meet the unique needs of Black male students, enhancing engagement and academic success.

3. Enhance Data Collection and Research:

- **Disaggregated Data:**

    o **Advanced Analytics:** AI can process large datasets to disaggregate health and education outcomes by race, gender, and socioeconomic status, identifying specific disparities and informing targeted interventions.

- **Community-Based Research:**

    o **Participatory AI Research:** Engage community members in AI research projects to ensure that the developed solutions are culturally relevant and address the unique challenges faced by Black men.

By thoughtfully integrating AI into these strategies, we can create more equitable systems that address the specific needs of Black men, ultimately improving health outcomes and reducing disparities.

Mapping the Opportunity Agenda for Black Men to the Social Drivers of Health Framework

At a high-level, an Opportunity Agenda for Black Men might look like the collective gathering of any interested stakeholders or any partners that are willing to work in solidarity to support this work where it aligns. This alignment supports the five components of the Social Drivers of Health Framework and additional opportunities discussed below.

Key Components of the Five Social Drivers of Health Framework

1. Economic Stability

- **Initiative**: Economic empowerment through proposed legislation, like a hypothetical *Black Entrepreneur Loan Forgiveness Act* and business grants for Black men referenced earlier.

- **Connection to SDOH**: Economic stability is foundational to long-term health and well-being. By fostering Black men's financial security and business growth, this agenda targets wealth disparities, creating opportunities that can influence household income, employment rates, and access to quality living conditions.

2. Education Access and Quality

- **Initiative**: Support for technical assistance and mentorship in business, as well as entrepreneurship training as stated earlier.

- **Connection to SDOH**: Access to business education and skill-building enables Black men to succeed in entrepreneurial pursuits and enhances job creation within communities.

Education directly affects future income potential and social mobility, providing individuals with the skills needed to build wealth and to improve health outcomes.

3. Healthcare Access, Broadband, and Quality

- **Initiative**: Improved access to substance abuse treatment and expansion of chronic disease prevention initiatives, such as those targeting diabetes and cardiovascular disease. Likewise, broadband should be recognized as a social determinant of health (SDOH) because it impacts various domains like education, employment, healthcare access, and access to credible information.

- **Connection to SDOH**: Health equity involves both access to preventive care and high-quality treatment options. By addressing barriers to healthcare services, especially in mental health and chronic disease prevention, this agenda aligns with equitable health access and strives to reduce disparities in health outcomes among Black men.

4. Neighborhood and Built Environment

- **Initiative**: Promotion of community-based physical activity and nutrition programs, alongside affordable and safe housing access. Collaborate with policymakers and health departments to support Black men who live near industrial plants, highways, landfills, and other environmental hazards, as there can be increased chances of getting disease such as cancer and asthma. Also, pay attention to urban heat centers in the city because a lack of trees can increase exposure to high temperatures in the community, especially during the summer. Therefore, there should be a planting of trees campaign. Additionally, climate change will need to be paid attention to as it can physically and financially impact vulnerable communities, such as increasing electric and gas bills during winter and summer months due to increased use of heating, ventilation, and air conditioning (HVAC) systems.

- **Connection to SDOH**: Quality housing in safe, well-resourced neighborhoods has a direct impact on health[115]. Affordable, stable housing can prevent chronic stress, reduce exposure to environmental hazards, and enhance access to green spaces and recreational facilities, which are essential for physical activity. This policy agenda would support initiatives that reduce housing discrimination, increase affordable housing options, and build communities that promote health.

5. Social and Community Context

- **Initiative**: Civic engagement, voting rights, and reducing barriers to voting for Black men.

- **Connection to SDOH**: Social cohesion and civic engagement contribute to community health and empowerment. By strengthening Black men's roles in the democratic process, the agenda fosters social support networks and promotes representation in policy decisions that impact their lives. This also encourages community trust and participation, both vital for achieving health equity.

Each of these components underscores a holistic approach to health, addressing social and structural factors that impact Black men's health and creating a framework for achieving equity across multiple dimensions of well-being.

Entrepreneurship Support: Expanding Access to Funding, Education, and Capital for Black Men

To foster sustainable economic mobility, it is critical to not only encourage Black men in starting and growing businesses but also to

---

115   The Relationship of Housing and Population Health: A 30-Year Retrospective Analysis

equip them with the necessary financial education, resources, and access to capital. Entrepreneurship support must be intentionally designed to remove systemic barriers and create pathways for lasting success.

Expand Financial Education Opportunities:

Offer financial literacy programs tailored to entrepreneurs, covering topics like business planning, managing cash flow, accessing credit, understanding equity financing, preparing for grant applications, and navigating venture capital. Partner with community colleges, Historically Black Colleges and Universities (HBCUs), Small Business Development Centers (SBDCs), and nonprofits like Operation HOPE to deliver accessible, culturally-relevant financial education workshops both virtually and in person.

Types of Funding and How It Can Work

Black male entrepreneurs often face exclusion from traditional financing. To close this gap, provide access to a diverse range of funding types, including:

- **Microgrants and Microloans**: Small-dollar grants and loans with simplified applications and flexible repayment terms (e.g., Kiva loans, Local Initiatives Support Corporation grants).

- **Forgivable Loan Programs**: Loans that are forgiven after certain milestones like job creation, business longevity, or community impact (e.g., New Market Tax Credit-supported funds, emerging models like the proposed *Black Entrepreneur Loan Forgiveness Act.*

- **Crowdfunding Platforms**: Training and support to leverage platforms like IFundWomen of Color, Kickstarter, or GoFundMe for capital raising.

- **Angel Investor Networks and VC Funds**: Connection to Black-led or equity-focused investment networks such as Harlem Capital, Fearless Fund, or Collab Capital.

- **Government Funding Resources**: Education on navigating federal, state, and local opportunities like SBA 7(a) loans, Community Advantage loans, Minority Business Development Agency (MBDA) grants, and state-specific grant competitions.

Resources and Ecosystem Development

Build an ecosystem of support that includes:

- **Mentorship Networks**: Pair Black men with successful entrepreneurs and business development coaches (e.g., through National Urban League Entrepreneurship Centers, Black Chamber of Commerce initiatives, Black Executive Men Community, Monumental Men's Network).

- **Technical Assistance Programs**: Offer workshops on marketing, accounting, legal structure, procurement opportunities, and preparing for government contracting.

- **Shared Workspaces and Incubators**: Create access to low-cost coworking spaces, accelerators, and incubators that provide infrastructure and networking opportunities (e.g., programs like Black Innovation Alliance and DigitalUndivided).

- **Capital Readiness Initiatives**: Help entrepreneurs strengthen their business credit profiles, prepare grant and loan applications, and present to investors with confidence.

Strategic Partnerships

Collaborate with banks, CDFIs (Community Development Financial Institutions), corporate social responsibility (CSR) initiatives, and foundations focused on closing the racial wealth gap to provide funding, mentorship, and technical support.

A Strengths-based Approach to Black Male Societal Contributions

Black Men as Leaders in Health and Medicine

Black men have a long history of transforming healthcare systems and advocating for better health outcomes in their communities. From the pioneering work of Dr. Charles Drew in blood transfusion technology to contemporary leaders like Dr. David Satcher in health equity advocacy, Black men have made critical advancements in medicine, public health, and community care.

Despite being underrepresented in healthcare professions, Black men continue to lead groundbreaking work in:

- **Medicine & Public Health:** Expanding culturally humble care, increasing Black representation in healthcare, and advancing research on racial health disparities.
- **Mental Health Advocacy:** Addressing stigma, launching healing circles, and expanding access to therapy for Black men and boys.
- **Dental and Oral Health:** Increasing awareness and access to preventive care in underserved communities.
- **Health Innovation & AI/ML:** Leading AI-driven solutions to reduce healthcare bias and improve personalized treatments.

Black Men as Economic and Policy Innovators

Economic stability is a key determinant of health, and Black men have continuously broken barriers in entrepreneurship, workforce development, and wealth-building.

- **Entrepreneurship & Wealth-Building:** Black men lead thriving businesses in healthcare, tech, finance, and real estate—creating jobs, economic opportunity, and community wealth.

- **Policy Leadership:** Black men in government, advocacy, and grassroots organizing are shaping policies that expand access to healthcare, housing, and education for all.

- **Education & Mentorship:** Black male educators, researchers, and mentors play a crucial role in shaping the next generation, particularly in Science, Technology, Engineering, Arts, Mathematics (STEAM) and healthcare fields.

Black Men as Caregivers & Family Anchors

The stereotype of the absent Black father is disproved by research. Black fathers are among the most engaged in their children's lives, demonstrating high levels of involvement in education, caregiving, and daily activities.

- **Fatherhood & Family Stability:** Black men are actively shaping family well-being, advocating for policies that support paid leave, financial stability, and positive parenting.

- **Community Care & Intergenerational Support:** Black men play central roles in faith-based organizations, civic groups, and social movements dedicated to health, housing, and youth development.

Black Men as Advocates for Civic Engagement & Justice

Civic engagement is a crucial determinant of health, and Black men have been at the forefront of advocating for voting rights, criminal justice reform, and social change.

- **Electoral & Policy Advocacy:** Black men have driven landmark policy changes at the local, state, and federal levels, ensuring equitable access to resources and rights.

- **Violence Prevention & Community Healing:** Through mentorship programs, gun violence prevention initiatives, and restorative justice work, Black men have been leading efforts to heal and strengthen communities.

A Call to Action: Elevating the Contributions of Black Men

The John Henry Health Equity Playbook is not just a policy guide, it is a declaration of the immense value Black men bring to the health and well-being of our society. By centering Black men's aspirations and strengths, that include:

1. **Investing in their leadership** through funding, mentorship, and representation in healthcare, policy, and business.
2. **Supporting their well-being** by ensuring access to equitable healthcare, economic mobility, and educational opportunities.
3. **Amplifying their voices** in policy, research, and media to shift narratives from deficit-based to asset-based.

The following prospectus outlines a detailed investment strategy to operationalize *The John Henry Health Equity Playbook*, delivering measurable social and economic returns.

John Henry Health Equity Investment Prospectus

1. Executive Summary

The John Henry Health Equity Playbook presents a transformative, data-driven opportunity to close racial health and wealth gaps facing Black men in America. Through strategic investment in health access, economic mobility, and civic engagement, this initiative seeks to unlock billions in economic growth while delivering life-changing results for individuals and communities. Entities like the Black Executive Men Community or the Monumental Men's Network could potentially lead this effort.

Target Raise: $10 million over four years
Anticipated Returns:
* Economic ROI: $3–$5 for every $1 invested.
* Social ROI: Improved life expectancy, greater economic productivity, stronger communities

2. Investment Thesis

The economic cost of racial health disparities exceeds $421 billion annually with education-related disparities adding another $940 billion. Black men's health disparities contribute significantly to these losses. *The John Henry Health Equity Playbook* offers a timely solution to reverse these trends, yielding both economic and social returns.

3. Investment Pillars and Potential Financial Impact

Pillar	Investment Focus	Financial Returns
Health Equity	Expand healthcare access, mental health services, preventive care	Reduce $100M+ in healthcare costs
Economic Stability	Workforce development, business loan forgiveness, homeownership programs	Boost incomes, business ownership
Civic Empowerment	Voter mobilization, policy advocacy, fatherhood support	Secure $50M+ in public Investments

Note on Potential Impact Estimates

These estimates are directional and based on national research demonstrating the financial and social benefits of equity-focused investments:

- **Health Equity:** CDC and HHS prevention studies show every $1 invested in programs like hypertension control and mental health saves $3–$6 in medical costs.

- **Economic Stability:** McKinsey and Brookings research estimate closing the Black–white wealth gap could add $1–$1.5 trillion to U.S. GDP by 2028; targeted loan forgiveness, workforce development, and homeownership supports are proven pathways toward that goal.

- **Civic Empowerment:** Research from the NAACP Legal Defense Fund and Black Male Voter Project shows higher turnout in marginalized communities is directly linked to increased allocations of federal, state, and local funds for schools, healthcare, and infrastructure.

These are not precise forecasts but conservative illustrations of how targeted investments in Black men's health, wealth, and civic power can generate measurable returns for individuals, families, and society.

Health Equity Sidebar

Case Example: What $100M in Health Cost Savings Could Look Like

- **Mental Health Access:** Fund 200 community-based clinics with culturally competent counselors serving 50,000 Black men annually.
- **Chronic Disease Prevention:** Provide free hypertension screenings and follow-up care for 500,000 residents in high-risk neighborhoods.
- **Community Health Workers:** Train and employ 1,000 Black male community health workers—creating jobs and improving outcomes.
- **Hospital Savings:** Reduce uncompensated ER visits, freeing up tens of millions to reinvest in prevention.

Bottom line: $100M in savings = more clinics, more jobs, better access, stronger community resilience.

Economic Stability Sidebar

Case Example: What Economic Stability Investments Could Deliver

- **Workforce Development:** Train 10,000 Black men for careers in tech, healthcare, and trades.
- **Business Growth:** Forgive $50M in loans for Black-owned businesses, creating 15,000 jobs.
- **Homeownership:** Provide down payment support to 5,000 first-time Black male homebuyers.

- **Wealth Building:** Expand financial literacy for 25,000 Black men to grow savings and credit.

Bottom line: Closing wealth gaps fuels stronger families, thriving communities, and economic growth that benefits all.

Civic Empowerment Sidebar

Case Example: What $50M in Public Investments Could Mean Through Civic Power

- **Education:** Secure $20M in new funding for schools in Black neighborhoods.
- **Healthcare:** Direct $15M to expand mobile health clinics in underserved areas.
- **Infrastructure:** Win $10M for sidewalks, parks, and safe transit routes.
- **Fatherhood Support:** Invest $5M in programs for mentorship, workforce support, and parenting.

Bottom line: Civic engagement brings real returns in schools, healthcare, infrastructure, and family supports.

4. Key Impact Metrics (over four years)

* 5% decrease in Black male unemployment
* 25% growth in Black-owned businesses
* 15% increase in Black male homeownership
* 10% reduction in chronic disease mortality
* 20% increase in Black men's voter registration (ages 18–44)

5. Funding Allocation Area

	% of Total Investment
Health Equity	30%
Economic Mobility	40%
Civic Engagement	20%
Infrastructure & Evaluation	10%

6. Closing Call to Action

Investing in Black men's health and wealth is not just a moral imperative, it is a high-return opportunity. We invite you to partner with us to build a healthier, wealthier, and stronger future for America.

The Ripple Effect of Equity Investments

Research consistently shows that equity-focused investments deliver returns far beyond their target group:

- **Medicaid expansion** reduced mortality across all racial groups, especially in states that expanded coverage.
- **Father engagement programs** reduce incarceration rates and boost educational outcomes for children, regardless of race.
- **Community violence intervention programs** benefit entire neighborhoods, improving safety and economic mobility for all residents.
- **Culturally humble care models** improve patient satisfaction and reduce malpractice claims across racial groups.

Supporting Black men is a gateway to supporting society. Equity is not a zero-sum game. It is a multiplier of opportunity.

Legal Considerations for Policy Advocacy

The John Henry Health Equity Playbook is intended to inform, educate, and inspire only.

To stay compliant when advocating and/or lobbying:

- Focus on nonpartisan education and storytelling.
- Frame activities as community education, civic engagement, or awareness-building.
- For nonprofits: Use the 501(h) election to clarify allowable lobbying expenditures.
- When in doubt, consult legal counsel or Alliance for Justice's Bolder Advocacy resources.

A Policy Advocacy Framework: Navigating the Inside-outside Game

1. Understanding the Policy Landscape

- **Research and Analysis**:

  o Utilize GovTrack for real-time tracking of legislation and amendments.
  o Employ Ballotpedia for comprehensive election information and candidate data.
  o Access the Congressional Research Service for detailed policy reports.

- **Identify Stakeholders**:

  o Conduct a stakeholder mapping exercise to identify key policymakers and organizations.
  o Utilize tools like a Stakeholder Analysis Matrix to prioritize engagement efforts.
  o Engage local community organizations to gather diverse perspectives and build coalitions.

- **Policy Goals**:

  o Define specific policy goals using SMART goals and/or SMARTIE criteria (Strategic, Measurable, Ambitious, Realistic, Timebound, Inclusive, and Equitable).

  o Create a Policy Goal Worksheet to track progress and refine objectives.

  o Conduct SWOT analysis (Strengths, Weaknesses, Opportunities, Threats) to inform goal setting.

2. Building Advocacy Capacity

- **Training and Education**:

  o Host workshops on effective advocacy skills with guest speakers.

  o Use online platforms like Coursera or Udemy for advocacy training courses.

  o Implement a train-the-trainer model to build local advocacy capacity.

- **Engagement Strategies**:

  o Organize community forums and town halls to engage stakeholders.

  o Create a community engagement toolkit with best practices and resources.

  o Utilize various social media platforms (e.g., Bluesky, X, Mastodon, TikTok, Facebook, Instagram, LinkedIn) for outreach campaigns and information dissemination.

3. Crafting Your Advocacy Message

- **Message Development**:

  o Conduct audience analysis to tailor messages effectively.

o   Use tools like Canva for designing impactful visuals to support messaging.

o   Develop a message matrix to align different messages with various stakeholders.

- **Storytelling**:

    o   Collect personal stories and testimonials to humanize issues.

    o   Create short videos or infographics to share stories on social media.

    o   Utilize platforms like StoryCorps to document and share community narratives.

4. Engaging Policymakers

- **Building Relationships**:

    o   Create a database of key policymakers and their contact information.

    o   Schedule regular check-in meetings with legislators to discuss advocacy goals.

    o   Utilize networking events and conferences to connect with policymakers.

- **Lobbying**:

    o   Train advocates on effective lobbying techniques, including direct meetings and calls.

    o   Develop a lobbying toolkit with scripts and FAQs for advocates.

    o   Coordinate lobby days where advocates meet with multiple legislators.

- **Testimony and Public Comment**:

    o   Prepare advocates to deliver impactful public testimony at hearings.

- o Develop templates for submitting public comments on proposed regulations.
- o Host community forums to gather input for testimony and comments.

5. Leveraging Media and Public Relations

- **Media Engagement**:

  - o Create a media list of journalists covering health equity and related topics.
  - o Draft press releases and op-eds to share advocacy efforts with local media.
  - o Utilize platforms like Cision or Meltwater for media monitoring.
  - o Contact local television and radio stations for public service announcement (PSA) broadcasting spots.

- **Social Media Campaigns**:

  - o Develop a social media calendar to plan and schedule posts.
  - o Create specific hashtags to track campaign engagement.
  - o Use analytics tools (e.g., Hootsuite, Sprout Social) to measure campaign effectiveness.

6. Monitoring and Evaluation

- **Tracking Progress**:

  - o Utilize TrackBill or Quorum to monitor legislation and track policy changes.
  - o Set up regular review meetings to evaluate advocacy progress against goals.
  - o Employ evaluation frameworks (e.g., Logic Model) to assess the impact of advocacy strategies.

- **Feedback Mechanisms**:

  - o   Create online surveys using tools like SurveyMonkey to gather feedback from stakeholders.
  - o   Organize focus groups to discuss advocacy efforts and gather insights.
  - o   Implement feedback loops to continually improve advocacy strategies.

7. Shaping Policy for Mid-term Elections

- **Election Strategy**:

  - o   Develop a non-partisan voter education campaign utilizing flyers and social media.
  - o   Collaborate with organizations like the League of Women Voters for outreach efforts.
  - o   Utilize platforms like Vote411 to inform constituents about voting resources.

- **Candidate Forums**:

  - o   Host virtual and in-person forums to discuss policy priorities with candidates.
  - o   Develop a candidate questionnaire to assess their positions on key issues.
  - o   Utilize platforms like Zoom, YouTube or Facebook Live for broader reach.

- **Endorsements and Recommendations**:

  - o   Create a criteria checklist for candidate endorsements.
  - o   Develop voter guides that compare candidates' positions on relevant issues.
  - o   Utilize email newsletters to disseminate voter guides to supporters.

- **Mobilizing Voter Turnout**:

  o Implement peer-to-peer texting campaigns using tools like Hustle.
  o Organize phone banking sessions to remind constituents to vote.
  o Leverage community events to promote voter registration and turnout.

8. Long-Term Strategies for Sustained Advocacy

- **Establishing Coalitions**:

  o Identify and reach out to potential coalition partners with shared goals.
  o Create a coalition charter to outline shared objectives and responsibilities.
  o Use collaborative tools (e.g., Google Workspace, Slack) for ongoing communication.

- **Capacity Building**:

  o Develop mentorship programs to support emerging advocates.
  o Create training modules on specific advocacy skills for new leaders.
  o Utilize platforms like LinkedIn Learning for professional development resources.

- **Legislative Tracking**:

  o Maintain a legislative tracking system using tools like Quorum or LegiScan.
  o Set up alerts for relevant bills and legislative changes.
  o Conduct quarterly reviews of advocacy strategies based on legislative trends.

9. Tracking, Measuring, and Evaluating Advocacy Efforts

- **Establishing Key Performance Indicators (KPIs):**

  - Define specific KPIs for each advocacy goal to measure progress.
  - Examples of KPIs include the number of meetings held with policymakers, social media engagement rates, and the percentage increase in community awareness.

- **Monitoring Tools:**

  - Utilize project management tools like Asana or Trello to track advocacy activities and milestones.
  - Employ legislative tracking tools such as GovTrack, TrackBill, or Quorum to monitor relevant bills and legislative actions.
  - Set up Google Alerts for key terms related to advocacy goals to stay updated on media coverage and policy changes.

- **Data Collection Methods:**

  - Conduct surveys using platforms like SurveyMonkey to gather feedback from stakeholders and measure perceptions of advocacy efforts.
  - Use focus groups to gain qualitative insights into the effectiveness of messaging and community engagement strategies.
  - Implement tracking codes in digital communications (e.g., email campaigns, social media) to analyze engagement metrics.

- **Evaluation Frameworks:**

  - Utilize frameworks like the Logic Model to outline resources, activities, outputs, and expected outcomes of advocacy efforts.

- o Conduct regular evaluations using a Results-Based Accountability (RBA) approach to assess how well advocacy efforts are achieving intended results.
- o Incorporate a Before-and-After Study design to compare data pre- and post-advocacy interventions to measure impact.

- **Reporting and Feedback:**

- o Create quarterly reports summarizing advocacy activities, achievements, and challenges faced.
- o Share evaluation results with stakeholders and community members to maintain transparency and accountability.
- o Solicit feedback from advocates and community partners on evaluation findings to refine and improve future strategies.

- **Continuous Improvement:**

- o Establish a culture of continuous learning by regularly reviewing and updating advocacy strategies based on evaluation results.
- o Encourage reflection sessions among advocacy team members to discuss what worked, what did not work, and how to adapt moving forward.
- o Utilize lessons learned to inform future advocacy efforts and ensure they align with community needs and priorities.

A Very Practical Approach

1) Face-to-Face Engagement is Key

- Attend Town Halls and Public Events: Ask questions about Black men's health, healthcare disparities, and policies impacting communities of color.
- Visit Local and DC Offices: Schedule meetings with your Senator or Representative's office.
- Engage in "Mobile Offices" and Community Meetings: These are local meet-ups held by congressional staff.
- Attend Congressional Briefings and Events: Track events related to health equity and men's health to build visibility and credibility.

2) Make Six Calls a Day

Call BOTH the DC and Local Offices of:

- Your two U.S. Senators
- Your U.S. Representative

Why Calls Matter?

- Staffers track the top three most-called-about issues daily.

- Calls from Republicans outnumber Democrats four-to-one, influencing policy decisions.
- Numbers matter: 500 calls about Black men's health forces attention.

3) Effective Call Strategy

A) Ask for the Right Staffer

"Hi, I'd like to speak with the staffer who handles health policy."

B) Give Your Zip Code

Constituents get priority tracking.

C) Personalize It

"As a Black father, I'm concerned about healthcare access for Black men."

D) Focus on One or Two Issues Per Call

1) Health Equity and Black Men's Health: Support the Office of Men's Health.
2) Voting Rights: Protect Black civic engagement.

E) Be Clear and Direct

"I want Senator X to support legislation creating an Office of Men's Health."

F) Call Even if They Get Annoyed

Staffers turn over every six weeks. Consistency wins!

4) Organizing for Collective Impact

- Build a Call Squad: Recruit five friends to make daily calls.

- Use Social Media: Share call scripts and updates.
- Track Votes: Use GovTrack, OpenSecrets, or Quorum to monitor legislators.

5) Make Calls Easier with a System

- Save Their Numbers: Store as P – Politician for quick access.
- Set a Daily Reminder: Call at lunch or while commuting.
- Use Scripts: If nervous, follow a script.

Sample Call Script

For the Office of Men's Health:

"Hello, my name is [Your Name], and I am a constituent from [Your Zip Code]. I urge [Senator/Representative X] to support legislation creating an Office of Men's Health in HHS. Black men have the lowest life expectancy in the U.S. We need federal leadership to address disparities in heart disease, cancer, and mental health. Will [he/she/they] champion this issue?"

For Black Men's Voting Rights and Civic Engagement:

"Hello, my name is [Your Name], and I am calling from [Your Zip Code]. I urge [Senator/Representative X] to protect Black men's voting rights by supporting federal protections against voter suppression. Will [he/she/they] support this?"

Grassroots Fundraising Strategy –High-Conversion Potential

Step 1 – Prepare Your List

- Identify people in your contacts who are likely to be supportive (friends, family, community members, political allies).
- Tag or group them in your phone or a spreadsheet by shared geography, interest, or past political engagement.

Step 2 – Personalize Initial Outreach

- Send a short, friendly message asking if they would be open to supporting the candidate.
- Example:
  "Hi [Name]—I'm supporting [Candidate Name] because [one-sentence reason why]. Would you be open to getting the link to donate or volunteer?"

Step 3 – Share the Donation Link (with Disclaimer)

- If they say yes, reply with:
  "Thanks, [Name]! Here is the secure link to donate: [Candidate Donation URL]
  Paid for by [Campaign Committee Name]."
- Always include the official "Paid for by…" disclaimer if required by your jurisdiction.

Step 4 – Follow-Up & Track

- Make a quick note of who you have contacted and their response.
- Send a thank-you or campaign update to donors later to keep them engaged.

How to Advocate for Bills

Using the state of Maryland as an example, when there is a committee hearing on a bill scheduled, it is important to contact members of the committee. The General Assembly website lists all the committees, the members of each committee, and their contact information. Go to the main page (https://mgaleg.maryland.gov/mgawebsite) and click on the Committees tab.

Call or send an email to your legislators using the contact information found. Here is where you can find out who are your Delegates and Senator: https://mgaleg.maryland.gov/mgawebsite/Members/District. If you would like to include a short description of the bills, you can include the descriptions that are found online. You are also encouraged to include any details of why you think this bill is important.

Dear (legislator),

My name is _________________ and my address is _____________________. I am writing to let you know that the following bill(s) is(are) important to me and to all Marylanders. I would like to request that you be a champion for these bills and help get them passed quickly.

Each of these bills is important for Maryland, and I support them and would like your help in getting them passed. If you are not on the relevant committee, I would appreciate your voting for them during the session. If you are on the relevant committee, I hope you will fight for them and support the sponsors as much as possible.

Thank you for your consideration,

Name and contact information

Additional Resources

Practical Next Steps & Resources

(For Policymakers, Advocates, Community Leaders, and Every Reader Ready to Act)

The John Henry Health Equity Playbook contains a lot of information—and that is intentional. The challenges facing Black men's health are complex, and the solutions require bold, multi-level action. But reading alone will not close the gaps.

This section is designed to help you move from ideas to impact using the pillars, recommendations, and tools provided throughout this book.

Use it in two ways:

1. **Now**—to take immediate, tangible action within the next 30 days.
2. **Later**—as an ongoing reference whenever you revisit the playbook to plan campaigns, shape policy, or build community partnerships.

Starting with Small Wins

1. Quick-Start Checklist

Use this list to turn inspiration into momentum.

Step 1: Identify Your Priority Area(s)

- Choose **one recommendation** from each pillar:

  - *Pillar One: Physical & Mental Health*
  - *Pillar Two: Economic Stability, Housing & Education*
  - *Pillar Three: Civic Engagement, Violence Prevention, Fatherhood Support*

Step 2: Map Your Partners

- List **3–5 organizations or leaders** you can contact this month—think community-based organizations, policymakers, business leaders, or health professionals.

Step 3: Set a 30-Day Action Goal

- Examples: Host a voter registration event, co-sponsor a men's health fair, sign onto relevant legislation, or secure a meeting with a key policymaker.

2. Men's Health Equity Resource Bank

A starting list of national organizations, initiatives, and programs mentioned in this book:

- **100 Black Men of America**—Mentorship, health programs, and workforce readiness.
- **National Urban League**—Housing, entrepreneurship, and advocacy programs.
- **Black Economic Alliance**—Coalition promoting economic mobility for Black communities.
- **NAACP Legal Defense Fund**—Voting rights and policy advocacy.
- **Win With Black Men**—Civic engagement and policy leadership for Black men.

3. "If You Only Have an Hour" Guide

When time is short, focus on the essentials:

1. **Identify** your community's top three men's health or equity challenges.
2. **Match** each challenge with 1–2 policy recommendations from the Playbook.
3. **Find** the decision-maker or influencer with power to address the issue.
4. **Contact** them today — email, call, or request a meeting.
5. **Schedule** your next follow-up before the weekends.

Final Note

Change is not the result of one grand gesture, but of sustained, focused action. Use these tools to start small, build momentum, and invite others to join you. The John Henry story reminds us that determination is powerful — but when combined with strategy, collaboration, and persistence, it can be transformative.

Playbook Launch Campaign Prayer

As a man of deep faith, it is very important for me to give honor to my Lord and Savior Jesus Christ who made this all possible. This was my launch campaign prayer.

Heavenly Father,

I come before You with a heart full of gratitude and expectation. Thank You for the vision, wisdom, and purpose behind *The John Henry Health Equity Playbook*. Thank You for every experience, every lesson, and every person You have brought into this journey. I acknowledge that unless You build this house, I labor in vain (Psalm 127:1). So, I invite You fully into every part of this campaign—into every meeting, every decision, every event, every detail.

Prayer for Vision and Purpose

Thank You, Lord, for planting this vision deep within me. Let it remain rooted in justice, compassion, and truth. Use *The John Henry Health Equity Playbook* as a prophetic tool to uplift communities, especially Black men and boys, and to bring healing where systems have long caused harm. I declare Isaiah 61:1–3 over this work: *"The Spirit of the Lord GOD is upon me, because the LORD has anointed me to bring good news to the poor... to bind up the brokenhearted... to give them a crown of beauty instead of ashes, the oil of joy instead of mourning."*

Prayer for Strategy and Planning

Your Word says in Proverbs 16:3, *"Commit to the Lord whatever you do, and He will establish your plans."* So, I commit every part of this launch to You—budgeting, venue selection, speaker coordination, promotion, press, and programming. Give me divine insight and sharp execution. Remove confusion, miscommunication, and delay. Let each step be done with excellence and intention, reflecting the dignity of the people I serve.

Prayer for Team and Partnerships

Father, ordain the right partners, collaborators, and supporters for this mission. Surround me with people of integrity, wisdom, and shared purpose. As Your Word says in Ecclesiastes 4:9, *"Two are better than one, because they have a good return for their labor."* Bless every team member, vendor, donor, and volunteer. Let unity, trust, and clarity guide our work together.

Prayer for Protection and Endurance

Cover every part of this campaign under the blood of Jesus. Protect the logistics, the digital tools, the physical space, the finances—and my own mind, body, and spirit. When moments of discouragement or resistance arise, help me to stand firm on Your promises. As Isaiah 40:31 reminds me, *"They that wait upon the Lord shall renew their strength; they shall mount up with wings as eagles."* Give me supernatural endurance for this assignment.

Prayer for Impact and Transformation

Let this not just be an event but a movement. Let every page, every panel, every post, and every prayer stir something deep—in policy, in systems, and in hearts. May this playbook serve as a catalyst for transformation: shifting health systems, empowering fathers, restoring families, and confronting injustice. I declare Amos 5:24—"*Let justice roll on like a river, righteousness like a never-failing stream.*"

Prayer for Legacy and Multiplication

Lord, I pray that this work will bear fruit long after the launch—that it will bless generations. May its message be multiplied—locally, nationally, and globally. As Habakkuk 2:2 commands, "*Write the vision and make it plain, that he may run who reads it,*" I trust that You will send runners who carry this work forward. Use it to awaken, inspire, and build.

Closing Prayer

Thank You, Father, for being the Author and Finisher of my faith (Hebrews 12:2). Let *The John Henry Health Equity Playbook* campaign reflect Your glory from beginning to end. I declare that no weapon formed against this work shall prosper (Isaiah 54:17), and I trust that You are doing exceeding and abundantly more than I can ask or imagine (Ephesians 3:20). May Your Kingdom come, and Your will be done—through me, through this work, and in this moment.

In Jesus' Name I pray,

Amen.

Contributors

Okey K. Enyia, DrPH, MPH, Founder & CEO, Enyia Strategies

Séan Bennett, Co-founder & President, Collaborative Partnership Strategies

Greg Brisco, MBA, Founder, Humanize Generative AI

Kailah King-Collins, MPH, CHES, Founder of the Emerald Doula

Everytown for Gun Safety Support Fund

Kyle Gordon, MHA, Digital Health & Public Health Strategist

Michael P. Henson, MA, 1VET4ALLVETS, LLC

Ifeanyi Olele, MD, Founder of Genesis Psychiatric Solutions

Jason Ottley, PhD, Education Policy and Leadership

JJ Parker, MD, MS, Attending Physician, Division of Advanced General Pediatrics & Primary Care, Lurie Children's Hospital of Chicago; Assistant Professor, Department of Medicine and Pediatrics, Feinberg School of Medicine, Northwestern University

Winston W. Wright, MPH, BJC HealthCare; Brothers in Public Health

Author Bio - Dr. Okey K. Enyia

Dr. Okey K. Enyia is a nationally recognized health policy executive, government relations strategist, and scholar-activist who has spent his career championing equity at the intersection of policy, research, and lived experience. He is the Founder & CEO of Enyia Strategies, LLC, a health policy and advocacy consulting firm rooted in the belief that purpose must drive policy.

Dr. Enyia has served in the offices of three Members of Congress, where he helped shape legislation and strategy on health, education, foreign policy, civil rights, and social justice. His policy lens is deeply informed by a commitment to structural change, intergenerational healing, and the transformative power of community organizing.

He earned a Doctorate in Health Policy from The George Washington University School of Public Health, holds a Master of Public Health from Chicago State University, and a dual Bachelor of Science in Biology and Biochemistry from Lewis University. His peer-reviewed work has been published in *Health Affairs*, *Preventing Chronic Disease*, *Public Health Reports*, the *American Journal of Men's Health*, and the *Journal of the National Medical Association*, among other outlets.

With *The John Henry Health Equity Playbook: A Four-Year Health Policy Agenda for Black Men*, Dr. Enyia delivers more than a call to action—he offers a strategic roadmap that is both time-bound and intentionally fluid. Designed to meet readers wherever they are on the policy-shaping journey, the playbook lays the groundwork for scalable change. It provides a credible, phased framework with clear benchmarks—making it deeply actionable for policymakers, advocates, and funders seeking to drive meaningful impact.

The playbook also serves as an investment prospectus, articulating the economic imperative of advancing Black men's health. Dr. Enyia outlines the cost of inaction and the return on equity-driven investments—framing Black men not as deficits, but as brilliant and resilient catalysts for economic growth, innovation, and stronger communities.

He lives in Washington, DC with his wife and son and is a Life Member of Alpha Phi Alpha Fraternity, Inc.

From Legend to Liberation:
A Blueprint for Justice, Health, and Power

In *The John Henry Health Equity Playbook*, Dr. Okey K. Enyia delivers a groundbreaking call to action rooted in the enduring story of John Henry—the legendary steel-driving man whose unmatched strength symbolized resilience, sacrifice, and the burden of labor at the cost of his own life.

But John Henry was more than folklore. Decades later, researcher Dr. Sherman James providentially met John Henry Martin, a Black farmer in North Carolina whose life embodied that same relentless determination to provide for his family and secure dignity through ownership and hard work. His success came at a steep cost: arthritis, ulcers, and exhaustion from pushing his body beyond its limits. Martin's story became the catalyst for the John Henryism Hypothesis, which links the health toll of high-effort coping to the chronic conditions disproportionately borne by Black men.

Dr. Enyia contemporizes these lessons, presenting a bold, four-year agenda to dismantle structural barriers and advance the health and well-being of Black men today. With three strategic pillars—healthcare access, economic stability, and civic empowerment—this playbook turns legend into lived reality, data into direction, and purpose into policy. Through vivid storytelling woven alongside policy analysis, Dr. Enyia humanizes the data, connecting statistics to lived experiences and bringing to life the costs—and possibilities—of resilience.

Likewise, too often, men's health has been framed as separate from—or even in competition with—women's health, family well-being, or community progress. This playbook rejects that false dichotomy. Health is not a zero-sum game. Advancing men's health—especially the health of Black and Brown men—is not about taking away from others; it is about working in solidarity. When fathers, brothers, and sons are healthy—physically, mentally, financially, and emotionally—families are stronger, communities are safer, and public health systems are more resilient. Supporting men's health is a shared investment that benefits everyone.

This is more than a book, it is an investment prospectus for liberation. It outlines the tangible returns—reduced healthcare costs, stronger families, thriving communities, and generational wealth—that come when we center Black men in policy and practice. By mapping opportunity to measurable outcomes, *The John Henry Health Equity Playbook* offers both a moral and economic case for action.

Shaped by frameworks like the African American Male Theory, the Social Drivers of Health, and the Targeted Universalism Framework, this book challenges readers to reimagine what's possible when Black men are centered not as problems to be fixed but as assets to be invested in. Each pillar blends evidence with narrative—grounding policy recommendations in stories of Black men's lives, struggles, and triumphs—to ensure this playbook speaks not only to systems, but to souls.

Whether you are a policymaker, community leader, researcher, or advocate, *The John Henry Health Equity Playbook* equips you with the tools to create real, measurable change—and reminds us that resilience must be met with justice, opportunity, and systemic transformation. By humanizing the policy agenda through storytelling Dr. Enyia invites us to reimagine—and build—a future where Black men thrive in both health and power.

Join the movement. Shape the future. Build and advance the infrastructure for liberation.

www.ingramcontent.com/pod-product-compliance
Lightning Source LLC
Chambersburg PA
CBHW050010070726
47598CB00014B/395